To Improve Health and Health Care

Volume VI

Stephen L. Isaacs and
James R. Knickman, Editors
Foreword by Steven A. Schroeder

To Improve Health and Health Care

Volume VI

The Robert Wood Johnson
Foundation Anthology

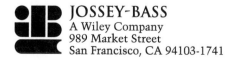
JOSSEY-BASS
A Wiley Company
989 Market Street
San Francisco, CA 94103-1741

Published by Jossey-Bass
A Wiley Imprint
989 Market Street, San Francisco, CA 94103-1741   www.josseybass.com

Jossey-Bass books and products are available through most bookstores. To contact Jossey-Bass directly call our Customer Care Department within the U.S. at 800-956-7739, outside the U.S. at 317-572-3986 or fax 317-572-4002.

Jossey-Bass also publishes its books in a variety of electronic formats. Some content that appears in print may not be available in electronic books.

Library of Congress Cataloging-in-Publication Data

To improve health and health care. Volume VI, The Robert Wood Johnson Foundation anthology / Stephen L. Isaacs and James R. Knickman, editors.
    p. cm.
    Includes bibliographical references and index.
    ISBN 0-7879-6311-9
    1. Public health—Research grants—United States. 2. Public health—United States—Endowments. 3. Medicine—Research grants—United States. I. Isaacs, Stephen L. II. Knickman, James. III. Robert Wood Johnson Foundation.

RA440.87.U6 T627 2002
362.1'0973—dc21   2002035657

FIRST EDITION
PB Printing   10 9 8 7 6 5 4 3 2 1

–ᴡ–Table of Contents

–ᴡ–Foreword

Since this volume of *The Robert Wood Johnson Foundation Anthology* contains Renie Schapiro's interview with me, I will keep my remarks in the Foreword brief.

At the Foundation, we have found a number of ways to "get the word out," in the phrasing of our former communications vice president, Frank Karel. Every year, we publish our *Annual Report,* which contains a message from the president of the Foundation, a listing and a brief description of our grants, and financial information. We also publish *Advances,* which, on a quarterly basis, offers the public brief highlights of our activities. Grant result reports and national program reports, which offer detailed analysis of specific programs and projects, are posted on the Foundation's Website. We're taking great pains to make our Website more accessible and informative.

Of course, *The Robert Wood Johnson Foundation Anthology* also appears yearly. Its editors have attempted the difficult task of combining incisive, unbiased analysis and high-quality writing in a single short volume that is useful to health professionals and easily accessible to the lay public.

I believe that foundations, as public trusts, have an obligation to be generous with the information they provide. There is probably no single best way to do this, but we at the Foundation are proud of our efforts to be transparent in sharing what we do, why we do it, and what we have learned.

Since I am stepping down as president and chief executive officer of the Foundation in December, this is the last *Anthology* Foreword that I will write. It has been my great privilege to serve in this position and to have been associated with so many significant programs, worthy activities, and remarkable people. My deep appreciation goes to all those individuals, many of them readers of or contributors to the *Anthology,* who have helped make these past twelve years so productive and enjoyable, and who have worked so hard to improve the health and health care of the American people.

Princeton, New Jersey   Steven A. Schroeder
August 2002   President and CEO
                                    The Robert Wood Johnson Foundation

–⚒–Editors' Introduction

The Robert Wood Johnson Foundation, which began operating as a national foundation in 1972 with a bequest from former Johnson & Johnson chairman Gen. Robert Wood Johnson valued at $1.2 billion, has grown into the nation's fifth-largest foundation, with assets of approximately $8 billion. It distributes nearly half a billion dollars annually, primarily in the form of grants to organizations carrying out demonstration projects, providing education and training, conducting communications activities, doing research, carrying out evaluations, and giving technical assistance.

To attain its mission of improving the health and health care of all Americans and reach its goals of (1) ensuring that all Americans have access to basic health care at a reasonable cost; (2) improving care and support for people with chronic health conditions; (3) promoting healthy communities and life styles; and (4) reducing the personal, social, and economic harm caused by substance abuse (tobacco, alcohol, and illicit drugs), the 245-person Foundation staff works along two parallel tracks.

One track focuses on improving *health care* (that is, medical services and coverage), with teams of staff members developing and funding programs on health insurance, management of specific illnesses, support services for people with chronic conditions, end-of-life care, and disadvantaged populations.

The other track focuses on improving *health,* with particular attention to the nonmedical factors that influence health. Teams of staff members develop and fund programs in these areas: alcohol and illegal drugs, tobacco, population health sciences, health and behavior, and community health.

The staff's recommendations for funding are transmitted to the board of trustees, which meets four times a year.

Sixty-eight percent of the Foundation's grant money goes to national programs that are carried out in numerous sites throughout the nation and managed by national program offices. Thirty-two percent goes to *ad hoc* programs, which are generally research, conferences, or demonstration projects carried out a single site.

At any given time, the Foundation manages roughly 2,500 grants. Just keeping track of this many projects—much less drawing lessons from them— is a mammoth undertaking. As Steven Schroeder observes in his Foreword to this *Anthology,* the Foundation has developed a number of ways to learn from its grants and grantees and to share information with the field and the public. One of them is the *Anthology,* in which we, as the series' editors, try to present a clear, unvarnished, and readable look at a range of Foundation programs. To do this, we recruit outstanding (often award-winning) journalists, program evaluators, national program officials, and Foundation staff members to write chapters. In addition, we attempt to demystify the world of philanthropy, at least as practiced by The Robert Wood Johnson Foundation, by asking staff members to reflect on why and how important decisions were made and priorities were determined.

This year's volume of the *Anthology* contains chapters on a variety of Foundation activities. It begins, in Section One, with an interview of Steven Schroeder by writer Renie Schapiro, in which the outgoing president and CEO reflects on the Foundation and, more generally, on health and health care since he became president in 1990.

It continues with three chapters in Section Two, "Improving Health Care," that examine the health care system and how to improve access to, and the quality of, health care. In Chapter Two, writer Carolyn Newbergh examines the Health Tracking initiative, a large-scale effort to understand the effect of market forces on access, quality, and cost. In Chapter Three, journalist and program evaluator Irene M. Wielawski writes about the Practice Sights initiative, a ten-state demonstration program to encourage health professionals to practice in underserved rural areas. Since the 1990s, the Foundation has made a major effort to improve the care seriously ill people receive toward the end of their lives; in Chapter Four, journalist Ethan Bronner analyzes the Foundation's strategies and investments to stimulate interest in and build this field.

In Section Three, "Improving Health," the *Anthology* explores how the Foundation has attempted to improve health by reducing smoking and alcohol abuse. In Chapter Five, author Digby Diehl looks at the National Center for Tobacco-Free Kids and its involvement in settlement negotiations with the tobacco companies. In Chapter Six, C. Tracy Orleans, a senior program officer and senior scientist at The Robert Wood Johnson Foundation, and journalist Joseph Alper combine to examine the Foundation's efforts to make tobacco cessation a part of normal medical practice. In Chapter Seven, author Paul Brodeur takes a close look at a single site in a national endeavor: the Fighting Back and Healthy Nations programs of Gallup, New Mexico. He tells the story of Gallup's efforts to fight alcohol abuse among Native Americans coming to town from the surrounding reservations.

The two chapters in Section Four look at programs designed to strengthen human capacity. In Chapter Eight, David C. Colby, a senior program officer at the Foundation, takes a retrospective look at its investments intended to interest social scientists in health policy and to increase their ability to conduct health policy analysis. In Chapter Nine, writer Paul Mantell describes another kind of program, The Robert Wood Johnson Community Health Leadership Program, that honors local leaders who have made a difference in their communities.

In this *Anthology*, as in previous volumes, we examine a major communications effort. In the single chapter of Section Five, journalist Susan B. Garland analyzes a major communications campaign that supported the work of the Covering Kids program to get families to sign up their children for health insurance coverage under a new program established by the federal government.

The *Anthology* concludes with a look back at a program the Foundation supported many years ago. In Section Six (and the final chapter), journalist Sharon Begley examines the "swing-bed program" (formally named the Rural Hospital Program of Extended Care Services), funded initially by the Foundation in 1981, in which rural hospitals converted some of their beds for use by patients needing long-term nursing care.

We sometimes refer to the *Anthology* as a public accounting of the Foundation's programmatic activities. We hope the series continues to serve as a public accounting and, as such, to be useful to those trying to improve health and health care as well as those attempting to understand the sometimes mysterious world of philanthropy.

San Francisco   Stephen L. Isaacs
Princeton, New Jersey   James R. Knickman
August 2002   Editors

—⚬—Acknowledgments

We wish to express our thanks to the many people whose efforts contributed to publication of this book. Our outside committee of reviewers—Susan Dentzer, Frank Karel, William Morrill, Patti Patrizi, and Jonathan Showstack—critically read every chapter; their insights greatly improved the final product. C. P. Crow, an extraordinarily gifted editor, strengthened the quality of the writing of every chapter. Molly McKaughan played a critical role as both a talented editor and a knowledgeable insider. David Morse made an invaluable contribution—twice—by reviewing drafts at an early stage and again shortly before the manuscript was sent to the publisher. Steven Schroeder and Lewis Sandy offered helpful comments on the entire manuscript. Michael Beachler, Alan Cohen, Ray Daw, Rosemary Gibson, Peter Goodwin, Robert Hughes, Paul Jellinek, Nancy Kaufman, Tony Kovner, Joe Marx, Maureen Michael, Dorianne Miller, Stuart Schear, Vicki Weisfeld, Judy Whang, and Warren Wood made useful suggestions on specific chapters.

In one of her first assignments at The Robert Wood Johnson Foundation, Ayorkor Gaba proved to be an able researcher in digging up materials on the topics for this year's *Anthology*. Hinda Greenberg, Kathryn Flatley, and Mary Beth Kren were able to find many difficult-to-locate documents. As in past years, Richard Toth and Julie Painter examined and corrected the numbers relating to The Robert Wood Johnson Foundation's grants. Ann Searight and Maureen Cozine did fine work in promoting the *Anthology*, as did Hope Woodhead, who makes sure the *Anthology* gets to the right people. Sherry DeMarchi was ever helpful, as she has been in past years, in a variety of administrative matters. Nancy Giordano has been a conscientious liaison between the editors and Frank Karel through December 2001 and with his successor, David Morse, thereafter.

Sara Wilkinson has been extremely competent and a pleasure to work with in her capacity as executive assistant to Steven Schroeder.

Paul Moran handled contractual and administrative matters at The Robert Wood Johnson Foundation in a professional manner. Tim Crowley ably assisted him. Carolyn Scholer, Mary Castria, and Carol Owle saw that financial matters went off without a hitch. At Health Policy Associates, Greta McKinney managed the finances and bookkeeping with great efficiency.

Lauren MacIntyre did an excellent job of entering editorial changes and putting them in a legible format. Charles Krezell did a fine job with the fact checking. At Jossey-Bass, Andy Pasternack has played a key role since the beginning in ensuring that the *Anthology* series meets the highest standards; Amy Scott and Gigi Mark handled the book's publication ably; and Jon Peck of Dovetail Publishing Services, with whom Jossey-Bass contracted to handle the print production, worked rapidly and thoroughly.

Two people deserve our special thanks. Since the first volume of the *Anthology* series, Deborah Malloy, administrative coordinator for the research and evaluation group, has been *the* critical person in making sure that communications between the two editors flow smoothly. She has always handled this task with great aplomb. Last year, Elizabeth Dawson, research and editorial associate at Health Policy Associates, stepped in toward the end of the process of putting the *Anthology* to bed. This year, she was involved from the beginning, and she has been a pleasure to work with, both professionally and personally. Our profound appreciation to both.

S.L.I. and J.R.K.

To Improve Health and Health Care

Volume VI

Reflections on Health, Philanthropy, and The Robert Wood Johnson Foundation

1

A Conversation with Steven A. Schroeder

Renie Schapiro

Editors' Introduction

Steven A. Schroeder retires as president and chief executive officer of The Robert Wood Johnson Foundation at the end of 2002. He will be succeeded by Dr. Risa Lavizzo-Mourey. An internist by training, Dr. Schroeder came to the Foundation in 1990 from the University of California at San Francisco, where he had been professor of medicine, medical director of a university-sponsored health maintenance organization, and founder of the Division of General Internal Medicine.

During his tenure, the Foundation's assets grew from $2.8 billion to approximately 8 billion, and the Foundation developed new programs to reduce substance abuse (particularly tobacco), improve care at the end of life, support coalitions of volunteers assisting homebound people, expand health insurance coverage for children, and promote physical activity. Under his guidance, in 1999 the Foundation was reorganized into two groups, one focusing on health care and the other on health. In response to the Foundation's growth, he also oversaw the renovation and expansion of its headquarters.

In this opening chapter, Renie Schapiro, a writer and consultant to The Robert Wood Johnson Foundation, conducts a wide-ranging interview with Dr. Schroeder. The chapter offers a rare opportunity for the chief executive of the Foundation, the nation's fifth largest, to reflect candidly on the issues faced by the Foundation over the past twelve years, and on the state of health and health care in America.

RS: Let's begin long before you came to The Robert Wood Johnson Foundation. What drew you to medicine and to the career choices you made along the way?

SAS: What drew me to medicine was a desire to do good, which came out of a family background steeped in humanism and social justice. I thought about law initially, but it is so tied to precedent and I was interested in mountain climbing and science fiction and wanted to try to deal with new, open areas. That led me to psychiatry, which seemed like a frontier in health. I was interested in people and behavior, and I thought that by being a psychiatrist I could tap into those interests. The other component of my career choices was that I wasn't a very disciplined student as a young boy, and I didn't shine in the sciences. So I thought I could dodge that hurdle by going into psychiatry.

RS: You ended up in internal medicine. What happened to psychiatry?

SAS: I had a very bad experience in my first class in medical school: I flunked my biochemistry midterm. It made me realize that I had to study harder. Once I started studying and coming back to the sciences, I realized that I liked them more than I had thought. So I saw other aspects of medicine as being possible. Then I took my psychiatry rotations during my third and fourth years of medical school, and the field just didn't fit with what I wanted to do. My interest morphed into how to combine medicine and public health.

On Coming to The Robert Wood Johnson Foundation

RS: You certainly did that. You have had experience in academic medicine, public health, and health policy, and as a Robert Wood Johnson Foundation grantee. How did that unusual combination of experiences affect your approach to the Foundation's presidency?

SAS: I was sort of a risky choice for the Foundation, because I hadn't had a lot of senior-level experience as a manager. I was medical director of two university-sponsored health maintenance organizations, and I had run a rather large academic division of general internal medicine, but a division within a department within a school is relatively low in the academic hierarchy. I had tried to understand clinical medicine; public health; and health care organization, finance, and policy, so I probably had more breadth than the average person in medicine. That kept me from being locked into any particular approach and left me with a sense that the Foundation should do whatever it takes to make things better in the broad scope of health and health care.

RS: In a sense, you represented a new generation of presidents. You are only the third person to hold the job. Your immediate predecessor, Lee Cluff, was from the inside and held it on an interim basis. Did you feel you were creating a template for the presidency of this organization?

SAS: To be frank, when I first got here, I worried that I was going to get fired. There was some tumult within the Foundation. I had heard that there was friction between board and staff, and I thought the agenda I was bringing was much more of a social activist one than the Foundation had seen previously. So I wasn't thinking nearly that grandly.

RS: When you first came, what did you hope to accomplish?

SAS: I said, "I want the best possible programs. I want this to be the best possible place to work." That's still true. I also wanted us to make a difference. I thought the Foundation probably hadn't linked up its moral capital sufficiently to a vision of where the country ought to be with health and health care. I wanted to revise our goal statements to have them be less about grantmaking areas and more about where the country should be.

We did that by establishing three goals. The first goal was to ensure access to basic health care for all Americans. The second was to improve the way people with chronic illness are treated in our health care system. The third was to reduce the harm caused by substance abuse. These were framed as social goals, and they furthered the Foundation's wonderful mission statement of "improving the health and health care of all Americans."

RS: Explain what you mean by *moral capital.*

SAS: I mean using the Foundation's reputation as an organization that is trying to make a positive difference. So if we say something is important, it may mean something. We've been told that the imprimatur of our name given to local organizations or people can be helpful. We do that, for example, in the Community Health Leadership Program and the Local Initiative Funding Partners Program, two programs that recognize local leaders. When we convene a group to tackle a problem, like the one we brought together to speak out on the need for broader health insurance coverage, that is drawing on our moral capital.

Another example of using moral capital—another way I've tried to say something is important—is by writing and speaking. By taking on subjects like the uninsured and substance abuse. I have not been as much of a public figure as others might have been, and that's partly personality. I don't particularly enjoy being in the public eye. And there's a fear that we are so big we might be viewed as being sort of a bully. So I've tried to use our influence but not overdo it.

On Grantmaking Strategies

RS: Let's talk a bit about grantmaking strategies. Given that your health services research was focused on effective use of health care resources and reining in profligate spending, it must be especially hard not to wonder if you are making the best use of the Foundation's money.

SAS: I think that's the major challenge in philanthropy at the end of the day: the nagging worry that you didn't do enough. It's a valid concern. I couldn't sit here and tell you that we've made the best possible use of the billions of dollars that we've spent.

RS: If you could start again, what would you do differently?

SAS: There's a tension in a philanthropy in trying to achieve your goals while also trying to work with your historical constituencies and to engage the interests of the staff, who come in with their own interests and needs. What I could have done is really start fresh in a certain direction. Other than believing we should grow the health portion—that is, the portion having to do with nonmedical factors such as smoking and drug abuse that affect people's health—I wasn't at all sure when I got here that I understood how philanthropy worked well enough to say, "Let's make a radical change." So our change has been incremental.

I probably could have been a tougher manager and said *no* more often to some of the grants. There were some grants the staff worked very hard on that weren't bad, but even though they weren't really terrific in my view I still signed off on them. I worried that the consequence of saying *no* more often is that you turn off the staff, and you need to give them the freedom to develop things. But in retrospect, perhaps I could be faulted for not being tough enough.

RS: Foundations can and do take various approaches in dividing up their money. Some endow institutions or make very large grants, some focus on a goal that's probably achievable and can be easily measured, others spread out hoping to hit a home run somewhere. Where does The Robert Wood Johnson Foundation fit on that continuum?

SAS: I've had the luxury of working here in a rising market, so we've had the privilege of having a pretty diverse set of strategies. The common wisdom in philanthropy is that the more focused, the better. The counterpressure is that interesting problems come up—bioterrorism, you name it—and so there's always a tendency to want to go after new things. I think my leadership style has been to try to keep a balance, both in the mixture of large and small grants and in the desire to focus and yet not be too rigid about it.

RS: You mentioned the endowment's growing so much. Does that change your strategy? Do you make larger grants because you have more money, or do you basically do more of the same?

SAS: That growth permitted us to fund some very large programs and to increase our priority on improving health, essentially from zero, without being seen as taking money away from our health care work, such as expanding health insurance coverage and improving care for people with chronic illnesses.

RS: What happens when you have expanded programs in place and the market drops?

SAS: We have a multiyear program planning and budgeting process, so we're well positioned to respond to market changes. I do believe that discipline is important. When times get harder, you have to see what your real priorities are and what would be nice to do this year but you can't—that's a very helpful exercise.

RS: What have you learned about philanthropies working together?

SAS: It isn't done nearly as often as it should be. That's related to the fact that the transaction costs are often great because each foundation has its own board and staff, culture, rules, and procedures. Our Local Initiative Funding Partners Program, which is larger now than when I got here, is probably a model for large foundations working with smaller ones. I don't think any other national philanthropy does that. We've been less successful in working with other large foundations—there are only a handful of examples where we've done it. I'm not proud of that.

RS: It's almost a cliché now that foundations can take risks and even fail sometimes. Yet foundations in general have a reputation for being pretty staid and not often out front. Why is that?

SAS: I think that the reluctance to take risks is mostly staff-driven, although trustees often get blamed for it. You get staff members coming to work for a foundation who are drawn by the mission; they want to do social good. They have to work with others, so it's very hard to measure how much good they've done and how much impact they've had as individuals. One way they can do it is to see how many of the programs they work on get funded. The riskier your program is, the harder the sell to your colleagues and the board; that's a disincentive to take risks. The other thing is that sometimes a risky program blows up. Then, of course, there's the question "Why did you support that, and what could you have seen coming?"

Boards can figure into this risk aversion, too. Some foundations' boards are drawn from people who, for a variety of reasons, don't want to take risks. There are many kinds of risk: of failure, of not making a difference, of controversy, of politics. When people talk about foundations being able to take risks, they're not very precise about what they mean. But with regard to really going out on a limb for a particular program, there's no question that the staff and the board—and the leaders—can be resistant.

RS: So it sounds as if "I'm willing to fail" and "Sometimes a program will blow up" haven't really been incorporated into the culture.

SAS: We talk about that. Once in a great while, we bring a program to the trustees that they don't like, and they turn it down. That actually happened to me once. I wanted to help the Chinese government develop a proposal to hold the World Conference on Tobacco OR Health in Beijing, and the board said no. At the staff debriefing later that day, I said to them, "Now I know how you feel."

There is this sense that being turned down is a terrible thing. It really shouldn't be. But it's very human for the staff to feel "I don't want to take that risk." Some are more comfortable doing it than others.

RS: Accountability has been a major concern of yours. What's the challenge there?

SAS: When I was in academic medicine, at the end of the year I could give myself and our academic unit letter grades. How well have we done in getting research grants? getting papers in the respected journals? Did the faculty get promoted on schedule? How did we do in recruiting faculty? in the residency program? What was the fiscal bottom line on our patient care? What do patients think of us? How do we do as teachers? How did we do in getting grants? I could have a pretty accurate measure.

At the Foundation, we're trying to improve access to care, create better end-of-life care, reduce smoking, and the like. The results are hard to measure. Many factors contribute to the problems we are addressing. If things get better, do we take credit? If they get worse, do we say, "It would have been even worse if we hadn't acted?" So we do polls and do measurements and try to be as specific as possible on our grant strategies, but it is still hard to know how much impact we've had. Ultimately we're forced into word-of-mouth and a gut sense of how much we've been able to influence a particular field.

RS: Have you arrived at anything approaching a formula for which problems are susceptible to change and which are recalcitrant?

SAS: When we're deciding whether to fund a national program or enter a new area, we go through five steps (not necessarily in sequence). First, how important is the problem? Second, how could it be made better? Third, who is working on it? Fourth, what has been the experience of those working on it? And fifth, how does it fit with what we could do with our culture, with the talent that we have here, and with the amount of money that we have?

One realization I've come to is that we tend to overemphasize strategy and underemphasize execution. A key component of execution is leadership. The people we've picked to lead our big programs probably had more to do with their success or failure than the very elegant strategy that we may dream up here. I think that we sometimes get ourselves into a box by either overpromising when we develop a program—that is, we oversell it—or, conversely, by being so vague that at the end of the day we can't really tell whether it did what we thought it was going to do.

But how to take a bite out of a problem is still pretty much an art form. One thing that we've done, particularly in health, is to try to give more importance, more support, to an underdeveloped field. We've done that with substance abuse and care at the end of life; we're going to do it more with physical activity, and to some extent with public health. The Foundation can support people who are doing good work in an area and have good ideas about how to make things better. That's been easier in health than in health care, because it's a less crowded field.

RS: Have you changed your notions of grantmaking strategy over your twelve years?

SAS: I've come to rely less on academics as a stimulus for social change. It's much more obvious to me now that grassroots movements and the media and politics are very, very critical. At least in the era since I've been here, academic medicine has been much more reactive than proactive. So I guess I've looked elsewhere for solutions to some of our more difficult social problems.

RS: Do you come away from your experience here struck more by how much The Robert Wood Johnson Foundation can accomplish or by its limits?

SAS: Both. I think the integrity and the reputation of our Foundation are great. On the other hand, it is sobering to see that social change comes very hard. That doesn't mean it's not worth trying, but it is daunting.

RS: Does the Foundation do enough to build on its successes?

SAS: On the continuum of foundations that stay in too long and foundations that get out too quickly, we probably tend to stay more with things. Do we do all we can to harvest what works? No, of course not. But I don't think one could accuse us of being a hit-and-run philanthropy.

On Priority Areas

RS: Looking back at the Foundation's priority areas—access to care, substance abuse, chronic care, and the more recent focus on physical activity under health—how do you feel about those choices now?

SAS: I feel good about our goals. It's at the next level down that I think we need more work, and I hope that as the next president, Risa will be able to help us develop even better strategies and execution.

RS: I'd like to take you through the three priority areas—substance abuse, chronic care, and access to health care—that were established shortly after you arrived at the Foundation, and ask you to reflect on what you think the Foundation accomplished, what lessons were learned, where that field is now, and where it's headed. Let's start with substance abuse and what you think the Foundation's investments have yielded.

SAS: I think we helped to mainstream the field. Since we are one of several voices, it's hard to know how influential ours is. But I think that as a result of our efforts, more attention is being paid to the importance of substance abuse as a social issue that affects many parts of our life. Institutions we've supported, such as the National Center for Alcohol and Substance Abuse at Columbia University, the National Center for Tobacco-Free Kids, and Join Together, are speaking out on these issues.

There's more flexibility about alternatives to incarceration—for example, with young people who use drugs. I think we've effectively served as a counterforce to the tobacco industry. There's more support for efforts to reduce the harm from drinking and drug use. Because we've taken some of the stigma out of working in the substance abuse field and lent it some of our prestige, we've made it safer and more inviting for academic and social leaders to enter.

RS: What lessons do you take away about how to make progress in reducing the damage caused by substance abuse?

SAS: Strong, effective leadership at all levels is a critical, important lesson. Especially in the antitobacco world, we found that there were warring camps— it was a little bit like Beirut—with many well-intentioned people working very hard who didn't necessarily want to pull oars together at the same time and with the same strength. That hurts the effort. We were able to have some effect on this through our convening role, but not as much as would have been desirable. Particularly at the outset, there was a fair bit of jockeying for position, and dogmatism. You know: "My way is the right way." Probably that's a characteristic of this field.

A second lesson is that in a field as complicated as substance abuse, you're probably smart to go with multiple strategies, and we did that. We sponsored research, funded surveys, supported a Bill Moyers television special, and helped to start institutions and form state and local coalitions. What would have happened if we'd put the same resources into just one strategy? Since we didn't do so, it's hard to know. But I have a feeling that in social movements like this, it's useful to invest in a variety of strategies.

Another lesson is the difficulty of mobilizing grassroots organizations to speak on behalf of people who have been harmed by substance abuse. With important exceptions such as Mothers Against Drunk Driving and Students Against Drunk Driving, there's no group of people lobbying for them. One disappointment is that we haven't been able to kick off a movement of concerned people—relatives of people who died of smoking or whose lives have been destroyed by alcohol or drug abuse. We have tried, though maybe not robustly enough. It's hard for foundations to start a social movement.

RS: Finally, your assessment of where the field stands now, and where it's headed.

SAS: It's becoming more mainstream. There is an increasing realization that the dollars spent in treatment are not wasted, although I must say that there's still a deep skepticism about whether treatment's worth it. People don't see that substance abuse treatment is like lots of other chronic disease treatment. People don't grumble if diabetes or cancer aren't cured; they still think treatment is worthwhile. But they require a much higher standard of efficacy with substance abuse treatment. Still, the realization is growing, and there is less dependence on supply interdiction. There's also more appreciation that countermarketing, both with illicit drugs and tobacco, can be a very effective prevention strategy.

In alcohol, there have been some new ideas, such as the concept of secondhand drinking that Henry Wechsler of Harvard University has put forth with our support. The idea is that just as secondhand smoke does, drinking causes collateral damage to nondrinkers—for example, on college campuses, whether it's date rape, noise that disturbs studying, drunken driving, or vomiting on a roommate at the end of a binge night. There is the realization that binge drinking on college campuses is quite prevalent, which people haven't thought about much.

Where the field is headed is also tied to exciting new scientific work. Back in 1991, we said we're going to work on all types of substance abuse, without really understanding quite how much common central nervous system dopamine pathways and serotonin pathways are involved in addiction—

that there may be solutions or treatments common to various types of addiction. The neurotransmitter and brain chemistry changes that scientists are now documenting will influence the direction of the field. I think there is going to be exploration of methadone-like substitutes for cocaine, and for pharmacological treatment of both drinking and cocaine use that parallels the work with heroin and methadone.

RS:　Let's move on to chronic illness and what The Robert Wood Johnson Foundation has accomplished in that area.

SAS:　The highlight of our chronic illness work probably has been care at the end of life. It's almost a signature program for us. We funded a major study that showed, unfortunately, that terminally ill patients—even those who had signed a living will or health care proxy—were suffering needlessly. After that, we helped launch a movement to improve the situation. We've worked with others, such as the Soros Foundation, to raise public expectations about what care at the end of life should be—for example, that people shouldn't have to suffer great pain and that health care professionals, clergy, and families should be more sensitive to this. My guess is that the country will do better on care at the end of life, and that we can take some credit for it and feel good about our role.

In terms of quality of care—narrowing the gap between what we know works in chronic illness and what actually happens—I don't think we have had much of an impact yet. I'm very hopeful that our new work on improving the quality of care will make a difference.

In the supportive services area, our Partners in Caregiving program (which supports adult day centers) and our Faith in Action® program (which funds local religious groups to help chronically ill individuals) have the potential to bolster a community support system and allow people to stay in their home longer, rather than go into a nursing home. That's what most people want, so I think we've made a contribution there, too.

But we've probably accomplished less in chronic care than in the two other priority areas, substance abuse and access to health care services. In terms of quality, compassion, and efficiency, as good as our system is, it could be much better. The problem is, it's tough making it better because there is so much noise in the system—so many people and players and so much money. The Foundation has much less leverage.

RS: How do you get consumers to demand better chronic care?

SAS: It's easier to get outraged about, say, smoking, because there's an industry that's pushing a product that's harmful and whose tactics over the years have been very deceptive. It's harder to feel outrage about your doctors or your nurses or your hospital, because much of what they do is wonderful.

So you tend to see family members or survivors advocating around a specific disease, and what they generally want is a bigger piece of the pie. The collective message from those voices is just "More for everyone," and the louder the voice, the better the chance you have. One of the problems is that people with chronic illness are not liable to be heard as much in the political process. Ultimately, I think the system is not going to get better until the customers and the people working in the field want it to.

RS: Let's move on to access to care. The issue of medical coverage has been a passion of yours. You've spoken about the immorality of having so many uninsured in this country. Yet the problem isn't going away.

SAS: It sure isn't.

RS: Are you discouraged?

SAS: I'm generally a glass-half-full person, but I must say that it's disappointing to see the lack of interest, both at the political level and in the health professions. In general, the leadership from medicine and nursing hasn't been there on this issue. On the positive side, support may be coming from some unexpected places—such as AARP [American Association of Retired Persons]. Even though most of the members have Medicare coverage, AARP's president, Bill Novelli, has said that coverage is an important issue for the organization because inadequate coverage earlier in life makes for less healthy older people.

RS: What's it going to take to change the situation?

SAS: I'm not sure I know. Cost containment and the focus on medical expenditures have been so distracting and consuming that the health professions have not been able to work in a concerted way for more noble causes. On the other hand, they didn't work much for them earlier, either. So maybe it's too much to expect that professions or industries will do something other than argue in their own self-interest—although I would say it is in their self-interest to have everybody covered.

I think one of the unattractive aspects of our country is the relative lack of concern about the less fortunate. From time to time, I've wondered whether we should get out of the business of trying to expand health care coverage. Then I ask myself, "What kind of a signal would it send if the nation's largest philanthropy in health and health care gave up on trying to make sure that people have health insurance?" So we've stayed in. I think we've done some very good work, but frankly, we haven't had either the creativity or the muscle to bring about change. Nonetheless, it remains a strong commitment for the Foundation.

RS: That brings up the tough period in the Foundation's history when it was linked with the Clinton plan. How do you look at that now?

SAS: Well, I learned that I was very naive about how the political process worked. From my standpoint, I thought, "Here's our new president; he and his wife are going to try to make a health plan. She doesn't have a lot of experience in health care. They asked us to help them to better understand the field." And our board, which had mainly Republicans, said the Foundation should help. We agreed to fund four regional meetings on health reform—"listening sessions." But in the execution of these meetings, I don't think we were nearly sensitive enough to the political nuances. So we were criticized, probably appropriately.

RS: What do you mean by not "sensitive enough to the political nuances"?

SAS: What happened is that the meetings became media events, with Mrs. Clinton being the focus, which elevated her profile and, by inference, her party. I sent transcripts of the four meetings to some people who had been critical of us for what they said was support of the Clinton health plan. Of course, those meetings took place as the task force was getting started, so there wasn't a Clinton health plan yet. When our critics read the transcripts, they stopped talking about that, because the transcripts themselves are quite innocent. But I don't think we were nearly sensitive enough to how it was going to play. We should be criticized for our naiveté.

What sobered me in the four listening sessions was the sense that everybody wanted more of everything and nobody was willing to say what there should be less of. At the end of those sessions, I went away pretty much convinced that we weren't going to get a national health plan—that the Clinton administration wasn't going to be as successful in achieving that as many people thought then.

RS: What about roads not taken during your tenure?

SAS: Two health care areas that we could have taken on more frontally are cost and quality. Costs were sort of an early semi-goal. We've helped support some of the intellectual work on costs—such as research done by Jack Wennberg and his group at Dartmouth that showed how much medical costs varied regionally—but it's very hard, in my view, for us to be a player in keeping costs down. So many forces are beyond our reach; we don't influence how payments get set, or supply or demand. Yet, without some control of costs, we're never going to get on top of access.

We were also concerned early on with improving quality of care. The field was quite fragmented, with a limited number of dominant leaders having different views of the right strategy to make quality better. So we went at it indirectly, choosing to focus on improving the quality of chronic care. It looks as if we are moving quality and chronic care together; my guess is that the natural trend is to link them more closely.

On Staffing and Managing the Foundation

RS: You've said that one of your greatest sources of satisfaction at the University of California, San Francisco, was attracting good staff. Let's talk about your staffing philosophy here. Your predecessor, David Rogers, hired smart generalists and worked them hard for a few years, and then they moved on. Some of those people—Drew Altman, Bruce Vladeck, and Linda Aiken, to name a few—went on to assume leadership positions of other major organizations and agencies. You seem to hire more senior people and more specialists. Do you see this as more of a place for people to build and complete their career?

SAS: I realized quite early that the success of the programs was going to be a direct result of the quality of people working on them, and I wanted to get the best possible staff people and keep them growing and energized for as long as I felt the Foundation was getting value from them. I inherited a strong staff, but I think it's even stronger now. We've been very successful in recruiting high-quality people. I was fortunate to be here when our assets were growing so we could continue to bring in talented people.

We are more differentiated now than we were in the seventies, and we need some generalists and some specialists. What characterizes the staff members is that they're mission-driven and work very hard. They can and should disagree on strategies—we probably don't have as much disagreement as we should, though there's a fair bit of it—but no one questions motives, and there's a lot of respect for one another. It's not that we don't have our issues, but I think this is a good place to work and people recognize that.

What's been interesting is that we'll bring in someone with a background in X, but they'll get fascinated with Y. We give them that opportunity to work on Y. Very few people work in only one area. The danger of hiring specialists, of course, is that if we shift out of their area of expertise, their background doesn't necessarily fit. But we don't usually bring a specialist in unless it looks as though his or her field is going to be an enduring part of our programming. We bring in people at all points in their careers.

Because we are so much larger, there's been a devolution of management of the program to outside the office of the president. I feel that's appropriate.

RS: Does that devolution—now organizationally into two units, each with five teams—jeopardize the focus that you have said is so important?

SAS: Well, people speak differently on that. Some inside critics feel that ten teams are too many. As I look at the aim and the content of each team, the teams make a lot of sense to me. If you push me, I would say we could probably merge maybe one or two of the teams into others.

RS: Staff and grantees must wonder how your leaving might affect their work. Can you describe what changes might come with a new president? What is there about the institution that will endure?

SAS: A foundation is probably more sensitive to a change of leadership than most institutions, because of the difficulty in measuring a bottom line, and the fact that the power flows very directly from the board to the president to the staff. In that sense, a president has the potential to make a major difference in the direction of a foundation, and I've seen that with some foundations.

Having said that, I believe there's a lot of continuity in The Robert Wood Johnson Foundation. For example, our programs to increase access to care and to improve the health care workforce—as through our Clinical Scholars Program®, Health Policy Fellowships, and our programs to increase the diversity of the health care workforce—stretch back to the Foundation's beginning in 1972. The board has indicated it's pleased with the direction that the Foundation is going; they would like us to do better and be able to measure better how we are doing, but they have not indicated that they want any major changes. So my guess is that Risa, as the next president, will make some changes, but they'll be evolutionary rather than radical. But we'll see after she has a chance to survey the landscape.

Our mission—improving health and health care—is much more focused than that of other big foundations, and we are likely to stay in both. But I don't think that our priorities ought to be fixed in stone. Things change, opportunities change, problems change, so I would guess that Risa will take a hard look at what we're doing and work with the staff to explore possible new directions.

RS: The core commitments and values you developed lend some continuity, too, don't they?

SAS: Yes. Let me talk about those for a moment. One of the options I once floated to our board as a way to respond to the Foundation's growth was having a "subfoundation" off-site. A board member, David Clare, who had been the president of Johnson & Johnson, stressed to me the importance of the company's credo as a North Star for Johnson & Johnson employees. If you have people off-site, he said, you need a set of enduring values that they can come back to, and that got me thinking and talking, and ultimately it resulted in the core commitments and values.[1]

On Legacy

RS: Your imprint, your legacy: What do you see as the three or four most important changes you've shepherded?

SAS: From the inside, helping to get a national board of trustees. When I got here, I was the youngest of eighteen white males, all from the East Coast. We were ripe to move to a more national board. Second, improving the communication between our board and staff, in part by having the staff attend board meetings, and featuring them. I'm very proud of our staff, and I wanted to expose them as much as possible to the board, and give the board a good sense of how things work here. The third legacy is the high quality of the people we have here. And we've got a wonderful new building that houses the Foundation.

More important, though, is, What difference have we made with the billions of dollars that have been spent since I came here? I would identify probably four or five things.

Growing the health part of our mission was especially important. We established programs first in substance abuse, then to encourage physical activity, and more recently to bring about broader behavioral change. We've also helped to build the field of population health.

In health care, I think our staying the course—the Don Quixote, the Sisyphean course—of trying to get people covered with health insurance has been the right thing to do even though it's a tough battle. Taking the negative results of the SUPPORT study on improving end-of-life care and helping to mold that into the end-of-life movement is a legacy of the Foundation. Some of our work in quality of care that we're starting now may turn out to be a legacy. Faith in Action, our program to help religious organizations whose members provide supportive services to their chronically ill neighbors, clearly has the possibility of becoming a legacy too. We not only stayed the course with the minority health professional programs (which have come under so much fire in some quarters), we've expanded them.

But I don't think of these accomplishments as my personal legacy; I think of them as a legacy of my era here, which is different.

RS: Is there a particular accomplishment, a particular grant, a particular change that has given you the greatest personal satisfaction?

SAS: The Foundation's work on smoking is near and dear to my heart, because tobacco is such a huge health hazard and philanthropy was conspicuously silent about it. I've felt that it was something we should be doing, and we now have a strong presence in the field.

RS: What was most disheartening or disappointing?

SAS: That we have more people uninsured now than we did when I got here. It's a double-barreled disappointment. It demonstrates to me daily the limits of what we can do as a foundation. It also illustrates the less desirable qualities of our country.

RS: You did a listening tour when you first assumed the presidency. If Risa does that, what is she going to hear?

SAS: I'm not sure. One of the dangers of a job like mine is that you don't always get the truth. People often tell you what they think you would like to hear, or they sort of lobby you. It's very hard to find a disinterested voice.

But I guess they would say that we could be more focused. Probably that we're more inbred than we should be, that we need to explore other grantees; we do tend to have a group of people whom we go back to often, because we think they're good, but also because we're comfortable with them.

They probably would say that our staff needs to continue to get out into the field as much as possible. I like to think that we are more customer-friendly with our grantees than we were, but I'm sure they would say that we could do better.

Then I suspect too that you'll get a variety of people pointing to what they think are our strongest programs and our opportunities for growth. To a large extent, that's a function of whom you talk with. When Lee Cluff took over as president, he sent a letter to a number of leaders in the field, saying, "I know you're a leader"—in mental illness or child health, let's say—"but knowing the Foundation's mission and what we've done in the past, all that we might do in the future, where do you think we should concentrate our efforts?" I looked at those documents when I got here, and found that people would rarely go beyond their own area. For example, the person with a background in mental illness would say, "Well, I think you should focus more on mental illness." As a result, when we looked at new areas when I got here, we did that as a staff function. We didn't use an outside task force.

RS: Do you come away from your time here with a different sense of what strategies work than the one you had in academia?

SAS: Convening, influencing public opinion, and social marketing are three very powerful tools that I didn't use much as an academic. I'm more impressed with what grassroots activism can do. For example, bone marrow transplantation for metastatic breast cancer was basically forced on commercial health insurers by grassroots advocacy groups at a time when there was no scientific evidence it was a useful treatment, and subsequent research indicated it isn't useful. That's a very powerful message.

My model of social change starts with the ballot and with campaign financing, which our Foundation can't do much about. If only 50 percent of the people in this country vote, and those who don't vote tend to be concentrated in poor and minority communities, then we shouldn't be surprised that they don't get as much from the system. So if I were reincarnated as a social change maven, I might work to try to get communities more active in expressing themselves politically.

RS: That's my next question. If you were starting your career again, what big lever for social change would you target?

SAS: I think we kid ourselves when we think that there is any one big lever. Social change is very hard work. The media—especially TV—has so much power, for better or worse. I would probably say—and I wouldn't have said this twelve years ago—that one of the most important people in our country right now is Oprah Winfrey. If you can get her to champion a social cause, then you have a very visible and influential advocate.

RS: How did you take that insight into the communications work the Foundation has done during your tenure?

SAS: We have expanded our communications activities significantly. We've supported some television and radio work, tried to create messages, looked to social marketing techniques, and supported advertisements about health insurance coverage, to give a few examples. We're more conscious of communications as a strategy.

On the Future

RS: What do you see as the major health issues in the coming years?

SAS: In health care, I see we're really in a box now. The clinical enterprise is growing by leaps and bounds, with the real promise of helping people lead longer, healthier, and more functional lives. But this comes at a great price. People don't want to be denied any access to medical care, but no one wants to pay for it. Politicians and the press are loathe to raise these kinds of issues. We've got about forty million people who don't have health insurance, and many others who are underinsured. So I see that as a collision course.

   In the health area, we're becoming more aware that many of the determinants of health lie outside the health care system. They depend on personal behavior. Yet we have a nation that's becoming more overweight and less physically active, and there's growing evidence that physical activity may be as important in preventing illness and improving functioning as not smoking. Trying to change personal behavior, however, is very, very hard.

We're also beginning to understand that being connected to one another may have an important role in health. All things being equal, people who are more extroverted and have more friends are likely to be healthier than people who are isolated in their community.

Another really tantalizing bit of information is that it looks as though relative income inequality may be a risk factor. It isn't how poor you are, but how *relatively* poor you are. People in the second quintile of wealth are less healthy than people in the first quintile, even though that second quintile is very comfortable. Researchers don't fully understand why, but they think it probably has to do with stress and the degree to which people feel in control of their lives.

So I see us sort of plunging down the health care technology track to try to make our lives healthier, while the real secret may lie elsewhere. On the other hand, when we get sick, we all want as much medical care as possible.

RS: What piece of advice are you going to whisper to your successor?

SAS: I would say things like I said in my "President's Message" in this year's *Annual Report*: mission matters; execution trumps strategy; you've got to know when to hold 'em and when to fold 'em; and don't underestimate the importance of leadership. I would say this is a very visible position, and people watch what you do. I discovered the symbolic power of what you do and say. So be a very self-aware leader.

Be as optimistic as possible. Try to listen really hard. A wise trustee told me quite early that you're not going to get criticized much, so if you hear some criticism, it's probably the tip of an iceberg and you should take it very, very seriously.

Challenge what's being done. Ask, "Why are we doing it?" "Could we do it better?"

RS: What are you going to be doing next?

SAS: I'm going back to the University of California, San Francisco faculty, as Distinguished Professor of Health and Health Care. I'm going to be working on a program with the Foundation related to tobacco and the health professions.

I'm on a number of interesting not-for-profit boards and hope to use them, and the experience and knowledge I've gained, to continue to be a voice for things that I care about.

RS: What if I told you that the board has just decided to move The Robert Wood Johnson Foundation to San Francisco and extend your contract? What would you do?

SAS: I would sigh! And I'd say, "Wow, that's very tempting." But I'm not leaving just because I want to go back to San Francisco. I really do feel that the renewal of an institution is very important. I worry that I might have gotten stale, or may be getting stale, or may become stale soon. I think there is a wonderful virtue to a foundation—to any kind of an organization—taking stock of itself periodically. The exit of a leader is a wonderful opportunity for that kind of self-assessment. But as much as I say that it's good to leave this kind of job, it's going to be painful, too.

Note

1. Dr. Schroeder set forth the Foundation's core values in his Foreword in *To Improve Health and Health Care 1998–1999: The Robert Wood Johnson Foundation Anthology* (Jossey-Bass, 1998).

Improving Health Care

2

The Health Tracking Initiative

Carolyn Newbergh

Editors' Introduction

The managed care revolution that swept through the health care industry in the 1990s was seen as potentially threatening or beneficial to some of The Robert Wood Johnson Foundation's most important goals. On the one hand, there was the possibility that capitated payments (set fees paid per person regardless of the amount of care provided) and discounted reimbursement mechanisms would impede access to, and reduce the quality of, care. On the other hand, there was the possibility that by focusing on prevention and coordinating care, managed care would improve access and quality.

Because of the importance of these issues, in the early 1990s the Foundation staff considered mounting a prospective "evaluation" to better understand this national experiment in market-driven health care reform and its effect on access, quality, and cost. The staff believed that such an evaluation could determine where the Foundation might be helpful in guiding or compensating for the managed care revolution.

More important, a careful assessment of the impact of health-system change could provide useful information to policy makers.

To undertake this assessment, the Foundation funded, in 1994, the Health Tracking initiative and created the Center for Studying Health System Change to run it. So far, the Foundation has invested more than $100 million in this ambitious program to help policy makers and the media understand the dynamics and effects of market-based health care.

This is not, of course, the Foundation's first involvement with managed care. In "The Changing Approach to Managed Care" in the 2001 edition of *The Robert Wood Johnson Foundation Anthology*, Janet Firshein and Lewis G. Sandy observed that the Foundation was an early supporter of the idea of managed care, then worked to improve standards for measuring and improving quality, and finally tried to smooth out some of managed care's rougher edges.[1] Nor is this the first time the Foundation has attempted to use research findings as a lever for policy or program action; in Chapter Six of this year's edition of the *Anthology*, C. Tracy Orleans and Joseph Alper write about an effort to translate research into action in the context of tobacco-cessation programs.

In this chapter, Carolyn Newbergh, a freelance journalist specializing in health care, examines the Health Tracking initiative. She explores the changes in the health care system and how the Center and its collaborators used surveys and other research methods to discover how the changes were affecting access, quality, and cost. She also explores the effect on Health Tracking when the consequences of the managed care revolution turned out not to be as dramatic as had been anticipated.

Newbergh does not shy away from exploring the difficult challenge faced by the Health Tracking initiative: to make its widely praised research findings available to the media and to policy makers in a clear and timely manner. This reflects the tension that sometimes appears between those doing research and those trying to communicate it. Resolving that tension is one of the keys to translating research into policy.

---

1. Firshein, J., and Sandy, L. "The Changing Approach to Managed Care." In *To Improve Health and Health Care 2001: The Robert Wood Johnson Foundation Anthology*. San Francisco: Jossey-Bass, 2001.

—w— The handwriting on the wall in the early 1990s wasn't pretty. Like an ominous EKG, health care insurance premiums had been rising at a double-digit pace as health care costs raced upward. Employers struggling to cope with a slow economy made it clear that they couldn't continue to absorb the increase in premiums. At the same time, the number of uninsured people was at thirty-four million and counting. Economic prognosticators were pessimistic about how we would get out of this fix.

Meanwhile, the Clinton administration's ambitious plan to reform the health care system, with its emphasis on managed care and competition, flatlined into history. Instead, the country was left with a de facto reform that was to be carried out by the private health insurance market. What was about to ensue was a virtual experiment in letting market forces try to come to grips with the complex system of private health financing and delivery, primarily through the mechanism of managed care.

Managed care held out great promise for making sense of the private system by instituting cost-containment strategies such as capitation, which provided doctors and hospitals with a fixed sum of money for a patient's overall care. This created an incentive to do only what was necessary for good care and not waste resources. Managed care was expected to reduce overuse in the system, which often saw too many unnecessary referrals to costly specialists or lengthy hospital stays. Managed care was also envisioned as using integrated delivery systems of doctors and hospitals caring for a specified population, applying medical practices that proved most effective. It was also expected to lead to more preventive health care, since physicians now had an economic self-interest in preventing illness and chronic conditions.

But as managed care plans began taking the place of fee-for-service insurance, the media were reporting horror stories: pinched-off access to specialists by doctors acting as gatekeepers to care; patients waiting for authorization before setting foot in an emergency room; and so-called drive-through deliveries, as women were forced to leave the hospital the day after giving birth.

What was truly happening? Were unnecessary costs being trimmed away and were the headlines just symptoms of a few growing pains as managed care evolved? Were premiums coming under control? Were patients getting more mammograms and blood glucose tests, or were they receiving less and poorer-quality care while being denied access to doctors when they truly needed them? Were doctors and hospitals cutting corners on care to reduce utilization and make sure the capitation fee covered their bottom line? What was happening to the uninsured in this climate?

Answers to such questions were hard to come by, because no one was collecting timely, reliable data on the private health care market's fluctuations. Government studies were often too outdated to grasp real-time needs; what's more, they had a national focus and did not target the health plan approaches emerging in local markets across the nation. Reports from private health care industry groups and analysts were driven by business interests with their own agendas, and these were often proprietary.

This glaring information gap was recognized during the days when the Clinton reform plan still looked possible. Many wondered then how to keep watch on what would develop. But with reform actually being carried out in an ad hoc way and heightened concern about its effect on the care patients received, the need for accurate, current information became even more pressing. How would anyone know how a market-based system of health care was working if no one was keeping tabs on this national experiment? Without a thorough, timely, unbiased source of information, it looked as though health policy decisions would be shaped more by anecdotes that grabbed media headlines (of the "Muncie Grandma Dies After Being Denied Operation" variety) than by thoughtful evaluation of what was truly happening.

—⚏— The Health Tracking Initiative Is Born

It was against this backdrop of a yawning information gap and the expectation of revolutionary change that The Robert Wood Johnson Foundation decided to mount a large-scale research program in 1994. Known as the Health Tracking initiative, the program set its sights on extremely broad and ambitious goals: to follow and assess the changes occurring in the private health care system, primarily in managed care, and what they meant to people. Health Tracking would focus, over time, on patients' access to care and its quality and cost in the many diverse health care markets in the country. Its hope was to generate high-quality objective data and analyses that would inform and thus guide the whole process of policy and organizational change.

This ambitious undertaking would have as its centerpiece the Center for Studying Health System Change, established in Washington, D.C., in 1995. The Center would oversee the Community Tracking Study, whose key element was a broad longitudinal survey of thirty-three thousand families in sixty communities, plus a national sampling. The locales, randomly selected to be representative nationally, would be revisited every two years to detect change and what it meant. The sixty thousand people to be interviewed over the telephone would be asked about their access to care, the medical services they used, their satisfaction, and their health status. The study would include two other surveys using the same communities: twelve thousand doctors would describe their changing practices and twenty thousand public and private employers would shed light on the kinds of health plans they offer and how much employees pay for coverage. Researchers would also conduct site visits at twelve of these communities for more in-depth interviews with up to ninety participants in a local private health care system—the major employers, health plans, safety net providers, hospitals, benefit consultants, medical groups, and consumers.

As it evolved, Health Tracking would add on a number of other outside "collaborative" studies to fill in the picture. In 1997, a study by RAND/UCLA would begin looking at access to substance abuse and mental health services in these communities. To better assess the quality of care being delivered, in 1998 a RAND Santa Monica study would start examining medical records in the twelve site-visit communities to look at a number of quality indicators. In 2000, a University of California, Berkeley, study would be commissioned to look at how medical group practices across the country manage treatment of chronic illness. The Foundation also added funding to provide small grants to encourage researchers in the field to use the data from the longitudinal survey, which is posted for public use at the Website of the Inter-University Consortium for Political and Social Research.

—∿—

Collaborative Studies in the Health Tracking Initiative

The lead organization in the Health Tracking initiative is the Center for Studying Health System Change, but other organizations also play a significant role. The RAND Corporation, the University of California, Berkeley, the University of California, Los Angeles, and the Research Triangle Institute received approximately $34 million to gather and analyze additional nationwide data about health systems change and its effect on health and health services.

The Community Tracking Study always intended to look at whether having a high level of managed care in a community makes a difference to people's health and the quality of medical care they receive. But this kind of research turned out to be so complex that it was spun off to consultants Beth McGlynn and Steven Asch at the RAND Corporation in Santa Monica. The study—believed to be the first population-based research that examines these critical questions—is expected to generate insights into who is at risk for poor health care and the kinds of measures that have been shown to improve quality. A sample of Community Tracking Study participants at the twelve site-visit locations are interviewed about their health histories, and their medical records are reviewed. The quality of their care is evaluated on the basis of more than one thousand indicators spanning acute care, prevention, and treatment of chronic conditions. The study takes into account income, insurance, age, gender, and geographic location.

The unbiased data the studies yielded could then be used for various purposes: to inform those responsible for health care policy at the local, state, and national levels about changes and when they might want to intervene; to dispel or confirm myths or anecdotes that too often drive health policy decision making, and to make a rich database available to the Foundation's own programs and health policy researchers everywhere.

This initiative seemed a good fit for The Robert Wood Johnson Foundation. The thinking was that creating better health care policy takes extremely good information. "Knowledge generation is a core strategy of the Foundation," said Foundation executive vice president Lewis G. Sandy. "The sharing of infor-

In another study meant to fill in the picture of American health care today, a team of researchers at UCLA/RAND is examining how managed care and public policy affect access, quality, and cost of care for people with alcohol, drug abuse, and mental health problems. The Healthcare for Communities Study, led by Kenneth Wells, Audrey Burnam, and Roland Sturm, looks at a segment of the Community Tracking Study participants intensively, with an emphasis on the poor and those at increased risk for these behavioral health problems. This study is compiling the first nationwide database on the behavioral health services that are available through public health managed care programs nationwide. Among the findings so far: most people with substance abuse go without care, most children and teenagers with mental health problems get no treatment, and just 30 percent of depressed or anxious adults receive the care they need.

At the University of California, Berkeley, a team headed by Stephen Shortell is examining how organizing physicians into group practices or independent practice associations affects their use of care management approaches for patients with four major chronic illnesses: asthma, congestive heart failure, depression, and diabetes. This is the first national study to investigate this linkage. Among the care management techniques looked at are use of evidence-based clinical practice guidelines, care-management systems, and disease-management programs. The study interviews physicians' organizations across the country, going into more depth in five of the Community Tracking Study locations. It also talks to trailblazers in using care management approaches. The hope is that the study will identify both impediments to managing chronic conditions within a group structure and successful approaches to managing patients' care.

mation leads those in the system to new dialogues, understandings, and potential policy choices based on what's happening in the environment."

To obtain such information, the Foundation had commissioned survey research in the past. Surveys conducted in 1976, 1982, 1986, and 1994 aimed at understanding the extent to which people had (and lacked) access to health care services. Every so often, surveys were done on how physicians' practices affected access and quality of care and the role of employers in private insurance. But it was hard to draw comparisons among these surveys because they examined different populations, were never linked, occurred irregularly, and were carried out by separate organizations with varying methods. Health Tracking was set up to eliminate those problems, by coordinating the studies and using the same communities and methods at regular intervals.

As envisioned, Health Tracking would be expensive (to date, the Foundation has committed more than $100 million to it) and time-consuming. The Foundation never spelled out how long Health Tracking would last. Many involved at its inception say they imagined it would function for at least a decade. Devoting such a large amount of money to research was rare for the Foundation. However, it has made similarly large investments in a number of programs that didn't involve research, such as Fighting Back,® Covering Kids and Families,® Clinical Scholars,® and Faith in Action.®

Any expensive, open-ended program, however, can invite criticism and even jealousy both from within and without, as this one has. Is it worth the money? Is it meeting the goals? The need to show results, to quickly find its place in the health care policy debate, has shaped Health Tracking almost from the start and continues to do so today.

—〰— The Initiative Unfolds

Recognizing that Health Tracking's effectiveness would depend on the credibility of the researchers who produced the work and the reputation of its organizational home, the Foundation approached Mathematica Policy Research, a respected consulting firm in Washington, D.C. To minimize startup costs and build on Mathematica's credibility, a new organization, the Center for Studying Health System Change, was established as a subsidiary of Mathematica. The Center began functioning in 1995 under the direction of Paul Ginsburg, a highly regarded health economist who had headed the Physician Payment Review Commission, which advised Congress on Medicare issues.

As its first endeavor, in 1995 the Center tested the Health Tracking concept through a pilot program, the Community Snapshots Project. Teams of researchers conducted local interviews and produced brief profiles or "snapshots" of health care developments in fifteen markets, selected to represent a range of regions, population sizes, and stages of development.[1]

The Center's first year of funding for the large-scale Community Tracking Study, also in 1995, went into planning the research design and startup.

The Center contracted with a number of organizations to collect data: Mathematica's survey group to conduct the household study; the Gallup Organization to interview doctors; and the RAND Corporation, through the research of Stephen Long and Susan Marquis, to study employers. The survey work began in the field in 1996. It took a full year to complete the sixty thousand interviews and three to six months more to put the information together so that it could be analyzed. This meant that a program funded in 1995 didn't start generating reports until the fall of 1997—a relatively rapid pace for traditional academic research, but a considerable wait for a center aiming at research that would plug into present-day needs.

Under pressure to produce reports quickly that would give the Center a public presence, Ginsburg, in the fall of 1996, began writing annual reports on costs, which were culled from his analysis of various outside sources. He was the first to note that managed care was truly leading to an era of lower premiums— a finding that was at first viewed with skepticism but that later, as the trend continued, gained wide acceptance.

Once researchers feasted their eyes on the first survey's data, they understood that they couldn't begin to describe health system change because the findings couldn't yet be compared with another period. "With a longitudinal study, you can't do more than establish a baseline after just one survey," said Robert G. Hughes, a Foundation vice president who helped spearhead Health Tracking. "The way the program is structured, the longer it goes, the more valuable the results will be."

What the program could do with its first survey results was to show what was going on right then, and to start debunking myths that had emerged. It was able to demonstrate, for example, that changes in health care varied from community to community and that managed care was not evolving to the same level of sophistication and restrictions everywhere, contrary to what had been thought. It also published reports looking at health care issues such as the number of uninsured across the country and whether consumers believed their doctors would refer them to a specialist if they needed one.

Even with this output, however, the pressure on the Center to produce more and to raise its public profile continued. After the second round of the household survey, undertaken in 1998 and 1999, the Center did begin generating reports, which started flowing in 2000. The reports showed, among their other findings, that slightly more families had a choice of health plan than two years before, and that the number of low-income uninsured children getting onto private health plans hadn't changed.

But then something occurred that had not been anticipated. The rapid, fundamental health system change the Center was set up to monitor wasn't materializing as envisioned. A curious thing had happened as health plans imposed restrictions on patients and doctors around the country: they balked. Angry about seeking authorization for a referral to a specialist and not being able to see a long-time doctor who wasn't in their provider network, patients complained to their employers, the media, and their lawmakers. As a result, legislation was enacted by many states and the federal government to protect consumers' interests. For their part, physicians were distressed about losing autonomy and income and gaining a mountainous amount of paperwork, so they banded together against capitation and for better fee arrangements. Hospitals, too, felt that care and their bottom line were being harmed by managed care; many of them consolidated and were able to use their greater bargaining power to negotiate improved contracts with health plans. Moreover, employers, contending with a tight labor market and eager to use generous benefits as a strategy for retaining workers, pushed insurers to relax restrictions on seeing specialists and to give patients greater choice of physicians and hospitals.

By the late 1990s, the backlash against managed care was in full swing. Under pressure from so many directions, health plans loosened many of the restrictions they had established to contain costs and to manage care. They eased up on barriers to seeing a specialist, gave their members a wider range of physician and hospital networks from which to choose, and began negotiating contracts more to doctors' and hospitals' liking. They also lessened or eliminated the financial incentives offered to physicians to reduce costs (and, some argued, to reduce care).

This meant that the very beast the Center was created to keep watch over had transformed itself into more of a mild-mannered, household pet. Fundamental change in the system was not continuing to unfold. Even the much-touted idea of creating integrated health care delivery systems of physicians and hospitals who would tend to a defined patient population—and would use an evidence-based medicine approach to their care—was not taking hold quickly. Most consumers seemed to feel battered by change in this period, but they probably felt it more as what news accounts called the "hassle factor" over difficulty in getting a referral or authorization for treatment and dealing with the health plans' bureaucracies.[2] Although, strictly managed care no longer threatened health care services, the milder version that had replaced it no longer held out much hope for stemming health care's rising costs.

Through its publications and conferences, the Center has been out front in describing the waning of tightly managed care and the concomitant rise in health care costs. In its September 2001 *Data Bulletin*, the Center was among the first to point out that premiums were on the double-digit rise again in 2001, up 11 percent—the highest increase since 1993—and would continue on this trajectory for some time.[3] Many similar findings came out through other organizations (business groups, consulting firms, and the government) during the following winter.

Sure, the Center was an important voice describing this retreat from tightly managed care. But if managed care no longer represented significant change, the Center's reason for being seemed to grow more uncertain. This put even more pressure on the Center to show that it was informing the public policy debate.

—ᴡ— Communicating the Research Findings

Once the Center began turning out findings, it (and The Robert Wood Johnson Foundation) learned the basic lesson that good research wouldn't get noticed without a well-oiled communications strategy. Communications would have to be given as much importance as the research itself if the Center were to become a resource for the outside policy world of local, state, and federal elected officials and their staffs; federal agencies working in health care; lobbyists; consumer groups; trade associations; advocacy groups; and academic institutes and think tanks.

Unfortunately, because of the way that the Foundation awarded the initial grant, the Center got off on the wrong foot in its public affairs operation. The original idea envisioned the Foundation itself handling all communications and being the voice of the Center. However, the Foundation later rejected this approach, and no money was allocated for communications when the Center was created. Many who were involved at the time say that the Foundation was uncomfortable with being so closely identified with the Center's findings, which might be controversial.

As a result, the Health Tracking surveys started out in early 1996 without having a public affairs approach in place. In fact, no funding was available for communications until July 1996, when the Foundation approved a $1.6 million supplemental grant and the Center hired outside contractors to prepare some publications and plan other dissemination and outreach activities. But this was six months into the first household survey, which was planned and carried out without sufficient emphasis on what would interest policy makers most. The Center's early journal articles and reports were criticized as wonky, dry, untimely, and not particularly relevant to the real world. At the same time, the Center was viewed as lacking in political savvy and out of touch with its audience's needs. Communication wasn't given its proper due until the decision was made in 1998 to hire an in-house communications specialist to coordinate a multifaceted public affairs approach.

Getting a grip on communications was critical because of the inherent tension between research and communications. Most researchers are by nature methodical, exacting, and cautious, and they are not inclined to rush their findings for the sake of publicity or informing the public. They often bury their findings late in a journal article after thorough analysis of statistics and previous studies. Generally, researchers are not of the rough-and-tumble political world, don't understand how it works, and don't put out feelers to see what people want to know. They achieve credibility by publishing their findings in peer-reviewed journals, which is valuable but time-consuming. For the Center, that added many months to the long process of generating results.

"So often with research, by the time it comes out, you're confirming the already known," one Washington health policy observer said. "It will have been written about in a less careful, less confirming way in the corporate press, but it's out there. And, in fact, a lot of decisions are made in the health care arena based not on careful data collection and analysis but on slipshod work."

Without a cohesive communications strategy, the Center missed opportunities to play a role in its early years, some say. One observer recalls that the Center sat on information that would have been pertinent to a congressional debate on uninsured children, saving it for a formal press conference the next week. "A more adroit operation might have said, 'We can tell you your numbers are off but we're not at liberty to comment further until our press conference,'" this observer confided. Someone else on the sidelines noted that the Center had to be pushed to think about how it could lend its voice to the Patients' Bill of Rights debate.

Once it hired public affairs specialist Ann Greiner in 1998, the Center focused on how to be relevant to its audience and reach out to it in a readable format. Greiner took soundings from policy makers about what they wanted to learn. Both she and Ginsburg worked with researchers as they designed their studies or looked at data to point out when something particularly interesting was lurking in a dense study.

To make its research more timely and useful, the Center began, in October 1999, to put out short takes on its findings in a four-page *Issue Brief* or a two-page *Data Bulletin* before a journal article is published. A number of journals agreed to this approach as long as the brief or bulletin mentioned where the subsequent longer, more complex article would appear. However, two of the nation's leading medical journals, the *New England Journal of Medicine* and the *Journal of the American Medical Association*, wouldn't go along with this approach.

Although the Center had employed these shorter publications before, it had never used them as a preview of a journal article. Doing so permitted the Center to gain recognition as a timely resource for health policy data.

Today, the Center puts out an *Issue Brief* or a *Data Bulletin* at least once a month and produces journal articles, *Community Reports* (from the site visits), *Tracking Reports*, and *Research Reports*. The Center also distributes press releases and briefs major news organizations before important findings are announced. It mounts well-regarded conferences three times a year on a current topic of interest and holds brown-bag lunches with policy makers to stay abreast of their interests and share the center's latest research findings. The Center remodeled its Website (www.hschange.org), which provides easy access to a great depth of materials. Media coverage of the Center's work has steadily grown, with more than one thousand citations in news articles during 2001. Ginsburg has become a regular resource for news stories on managed care and health care costs.

The Center also addressed one of its key problems: that a longitudinal survey is, by its nature, slow and cumbersome and takes considerable time to produce results. Because these surveys depend on repeating questions over the years to pick up change, researchers can't add and subtract too many questions from a survey without losing the ability to draw conclusions over time. Although the Center has made some modifications to the survey, it has learned to rely on site visits to the twelve communities that are studied in greater depth as a way to be more timely and flexible. At these site visits, researchers can plug in questions about current issues on short notice. They essentially take the pulse of the community and pick up on new trends and changes they didn't previously know about. "We see things at site visits that we haven't expected," Ginsburg said. "Our researchers saw network provider instability at a site visit." Doctors or hospitals were dropping out of a health plan's network, leaving patients to scramble to find a new provider whose services would be covered, or to pay more themselves for a doctor outside their network. "That was something we didn't foresee," Ginsburg added, "but we saw it so clearly that we could publish something before many other studies even began to look at it."

Some of those active in health care policy say they have been bombarded by Center materials in the last few years, and they like what they see. "In the last two years, the Center has kicked up its public persona in a major way," said Stuart Altman, a leading health policy expert and professor at Brandeis University's Heller School for Social Policy and Management. "I notice this in the amount of materials that it puts out and the timeliness of what it puts out."

Information coming out of the Center is now reaching a broader audience and attracting more attention, many said. "If I had to criticize the Center in the past, I would say the material it developed was not as user-friendly for outside organizations as it could have been," said Ronald Pollack, executive director of the advocacy group Families USA and a member of the Center's user advisory committee. "Over the past few years, the Center has really improved on that score very dramatically. Its materials are much more user friendly and it's cited much more frequently in the media. Organizations like ours find it much more useful." Within government, too, the change of approach has been noticed. "My health insurance staffers say the Center always has very well-written and easy-to-understand materials," said Richard Price, who heads a section of the Library of Congress Congressional Research Service that fields health policy questions from members of Congress; these questions often concern a specific district or state. "They like these materials because they keep them informed about trends in health care costs across the country."

Yet some staff members who support health-related committees said that the Center could do more to alert them about new research findings and reports. Others complained that the Center's work was still too slow to be folded into current political debate or to be relevant at all.

"I think they do very high-quality work," said David Nexon, staff director for health of the Senate Committee on Health, Education, Labor, and Pensions. "They could probably do a better job of publicizing what they do because it's tough to get people's attention up here on the Hill."

From another perspective, a staff member for the House Energy and Commerce Committee, Patrick Morrissey, said, "We have found them less useful because although we generally get their papers, there's not much follow-up."

In 2000, the Center sharpened its mission statement and reinvigorated its public affairs strategy for the coming years. It set a relevancy test for research, clearly spelling out that the foremost audience is policy makers. The Center commited itself "to strategically managing and disseminating its research for maximum policy impact." It set a goal of becoming the "leading health policy research organization devoted to understanding developments in health care markets and communities and the effect on people's health care." It also specified that its research would concentrate on three areas: private insurance coverage and costs, access to care by the uninsured, and managed care and markets.

To further these goals, when vice president Peter Kemper, who designed the Community Tracking Study, departed in 2001, the Center brought in Len M. Nichols, a former principal research associate at the Urban Institute, who also advised the Clinton administration on health care reform. Outside observers praised his appointment as being on the money, bringing the Center cachet because he is politically astute, knowledgeable about health policy, and plain-speaking.

Nichols said he planned to identify the health policy issues that were likely to emerge over the next six, twelve, eighteen, and twenty-four months to help researchers stay relevant. He will work with Ginsburg and Richard Sorian, who replaced Ann Greiner as public affairs director in early 2002, on early design of study projects, and he will make sure that policy implications are clearly drawn from research before it's written up.

"My job is to open a window into our own research and the general health economic and policy research so policy makers can get all they can out of us," Nichols said. "Then they can go into a room somewhere and do the playing, make the final decision."

—⟋⟍— The Center and Health Policy

Five years into Health Tracking, is this major undertaking helping to produce better health policy? Gauging the Center's influence on public policy decision making is complex. As many an organization that produces research has learned, the route it takes isn't easily traced; too many people read the information and use it in ways the authors may know nothing about. Having influence at all is tricky in a contentious policy environment of special interests and political ideologies, at a time when there is little passion for significant health policy legislation.

The Center can cite many instances when calling issues to the attention of policy makers has led to change or notice. Among them:

- After noting in a 1998 article published in the *Journal of the American Medical Association* that doctors who rely the most on managed care contracts provide less charity care, the Center was asked to present its findings to the Senate Finance Committee.

- In a 1999 *Issue Brief*, the Center showed that 20 percent of low-income people were offered health insurance coverage but didn't enroll because of the cost of their share of the premium. In direct response, the Senate proposed bills that would offer either a tax credit or a subsidy for workers to buy insurance through an employer.

- The Center's findings about the number of children who remain without health insurance, although they are eligible for the federally funded State Children's Health Insurance Program, was cited by senators as they proposed spending money for outreach to families.

- Two communities—Greenville, North Carolina, and Lansing, Michigan—strengthened their health care safety net after the reports by the Center revealed serious inadequacies.

The Center has frequently helped sort fact from fiction—for example, by finding that:

- Slightly more employees had a choice of health plans in 1999 than in 1997, contrary to the prevailing thought at the time.

- Surgeries and use of in-patient hospital and emergency care were about the same for HMO patients and those covered by other plans.

- People held negative opinions about managed care at the same time that they were satisfied with their own health care, raising questions about how to understand the results of patient satisfaction surveys.

The Center's work has appeared in more than two hundred of its own reports and journal articles, and the Website sees heavy traffic. Its publications have been praised as first-rate and its personnel as impressive. The information made available to the public has been requested ten times as much as any other Foundation data set. And in August 2002, *Modern Healthcare* listed Ginsberg among the "100 Most Powerful People in Healthcare."

Certainly, these are auspicious signs, but do they indicate that the Center has arrived at its destination? Is it recognized as a major supplier of high-quality, nonpartisan information that contributes to better decisions about health policy, particularly in Washington? Is it influencing policy makers' thinking?

Opinions vary, because these questions are difficult to answer. Perhaps the best yardstick for measuring the organization's effectiveness may be how it's regarded by the people it's trying to reach: the media and the policy environment itself.

News coverage is important to putting the Center's work on the nation's radar screens. Policy makers are inundated with reports they will never get to read, and news stories focus their attention on topics that matter to the public. When Ginsburg tells the *New York Times*, the *Washington Post*, or the *Wall Street Journal* that health insurance premiums are rising 11 percent largely because of hospital-related expenses—as he said in September 2001—he is shown to be a reliable, trusted source of analysis. Not only the public takes note; so do elected officials and others who try to sway the public.

"I turn to the Center because it's viewed as a credible source of information and nonpartisan," said Ron Winslow, a *Wall Street Journal* reporter. "They come closest to doing the kind of work journalists do in terms of gathering information about various communities and making assessments. So I think their methods are interesting and their information is very accessible to policy makers and to journalists."

Another Washington-based health reporter frequently relies on the Center for insight into "the economics behind the health care system mystery." This journalist praises the Center's output as top quality but laments that data are "not always as fresh as I'd like."

Staff members for Senate and House committees dealing with health policy and those in the research support offices for Congress couldn't recall instances when the Center's work had played a significant role in a specific piece of legislation. But many said that they and others in policy channels viewed the Center as a worthwhile, important resource, particularly useful for an overview when a topic is first being considered.

The late John Eisenberg, who headed the Agency for Healthcare Research and Quality at the Department of Health and Human Services before his death in 2002, said that his office had found the Center's studies informative; "Paul Ginsburg provides data of great value to policy makers that's complementary and not redundant to information we're collecting."

The Center's steadfast nonpartisan approach is an asset as well as a liability when it comes to impact, both staffers and advocacy groups said. On the one hand, the Center is producing sound, reliable information that no one else is—and it's needed to understand health care change around the country. "I think of them as one of a handful of groups that are unbiased, without an agenda to push," said one Congressional staff member. "You'd be hard-pressed to find anyone to say they're putting on a particular spin or angle."

On the other hand, not taking sides means that it's harder to get press coverage, and that policy makers don't look to you as often—and as a result, there may be fewer opportunities to be influential.

"Sometimes information that has a point of view makes it into the public policy debate, whereas information like this, which is more down the middle, doesn't," said another Congressional staff member. "This doesn't mean it's not as informative or not important to have the Center's kind of analysis. But when we're trying to develop a position or get quick support for a decision we've already developed, we tend to go to organizations that are more advocacy-oriented."

Staff members from a number of agencies said the Center's community survey data and market trend reports had found their way into their own reports—a sign that the Center's reach is expanding. "Our health insurance folks like these reports a great deal because they give them information no one else is providing, helping them understand very dynamic areas," said Richard Price, of the Congressional Research Service at the Library of Congress. "With this information, they're able to communicate analytically important information to members of Congress, the committee staff, and member staff."

Important trade associations increasingly issue news releases to highlight or respond to Center findings, and Center results are showing up in other organizations' own publications, which again suggests that the Center is gaining influence. "I find its products are fact-based," said Dr. Don Young, president of the Health Insurance Association of America. "The whole notion of being an early-warning system by looking at a select number of communities and doing it longitudinally is a very creative idea. Do we cite them, point to them as information on trends that are coming? The answer is yes."

Finally, being held in high esteem by other organizations suggests that the Center is finding its place on the map. "I think they're one of the few organizations that are really doing important work," said Karen Davis, president of the Commonwealth Fund. "The Center is up there with the top five or six places generating the important new information that's relevant to health policy issues."

—w— **The Future**

The Center was created to track major changes in the health care system; because they never completely occurred, questions about the Center's continuing role remain. However, as the Center itself has documented, the times ahead are expected to be increasingly turbulent.

Today, the employer-sponsored health care system is at another crossroads, much like the one the nation faced ten years ago. A double-digit rise in premiums is again with us as underlying health care costs continue to swell with the advent of new technologies and the expense of prescription drugs and hospital care. The economy entered a recession in 2001, and seven million more people were uninsured. Employers, feeling the pinch, protested once more that they could not afford to cover health insurance premium increases. This time, managed care is in no shape to come to the rescue. It's not likely to resurrect any of the cost-containing tools that were once so unpopular.

All signs point to a shifting of costs to consumers. Ginsburg and others have documented the fact that consumers have already begun to pick up the tab in higher copayments for a doctor's office visit and prescription medication, and more of this will probably be seen. But if consumers continue to be forced to foot the bill for higher costs, as expected, more of them will undoubtedly find they can no longer afford their health insurance and drop it.

Given that managed care's retreat is leading to higher costs and that there is great uncertainty ahead, a number of people within and outside the Foundation say that this is not the time to back away from tracking. They argue that the Center's contributions so far have been substantial, and that its analyses will be just as vital as they were five years ago—perhaps even more so.

In the meantime, after the Center's strategic planning process, the Foundation and the Center began to cut the cost and size of Health Tracking. Families will be interviewed for the longitudinal tracking survey every three years instead of biennially, and other adjustments are being made in related studies, amounting to an estimated cost savings of 25 percent. With health system change occurring more slowly, the Center says that not much will be lost in checking with the communities on a three-year cycle—and researchers will appreciate the less hectic pace. But the site visits will still occur every other year.

"The health care system is in worse shape now," Ginsburg said. "We have just as big a problem as when we started, but we have one less strategy. We can't see more than a couple of years ahead about what direction health care might go, because sharp changes are likely to generate their own backlash. To have the infrastructure to study changes, and the baseline data to do so, is a huge advantage."

Notes

1. Kaplan, M., and Goldberg, M. "The Media and Change in Health Systems." In *To Improve Health and Health Care 1997: The Robert Wood Johnson Foundation Anthology.* San Francisco: Jossey-Bass, 1997.
2. See, for example, Durkin, B. "Taking a 'Hassle' Out of Health Care: Some Plans Cut Referral Requirement." *Newsday*, May 31, 2000.
3. Strung, B., Ginsburg, P., and Gabel, J. "Tracking Health Care Costs: Hospital Care Key Cost Driver in 2000." *Data Bulletin* (Center for the Study of Health Systems Change) no. 21, revised Sept. 2001.

3

Practice Sights

State Primary Care Development Strategies

Irene M. Wielawski

Editors' Introduction

Since its establishment as a national philanthropy in 1972, The Robert Wood Johnson Foundation has consistently pursued the goal of increasing the access of all Americans to health care services. It has given a high priority to expanding the number of Americans having health insurance coverage—for example, by funding a series of surveys providing data on uninsured Americans, a variety of programs to make it easier for children to obtain health insurance, and a number of policy development and public education initiatives to keep health insurance coverage in the public eye.[1]

Insurance coverage is only one factor determining access to health care services, of course. Over the years, the Foundation has addressed a range of problems that hinder access. One area that has commanded particular attention is development of a health care workforce capable of providing, and willing to provide, services to people without a regular source of health care, especially those living in rural areas. The Foundation has endeavored to increase the number of physicians practicing primary care and has played an important role in developing the fields of nurse practitioner and physician assistant.[2] It has also funded programs to increase the number of minority physicians and other health practitioners, largely on the ground that they tend to serve minority patients.[3]

Beyond trying to increase the *supply* of health practitioners able to aid underserved populations, the Foundation has also sought ways to make the *distribution* of health practitioners more equitable. A major program to encourage health practitioners to work in rural areas was Practice Sights. In this chapter, Irene Wielawski, an award-winning journalist, the evaluator of the Foundation's Reach Out® program, and a frequent contributor to The Robert Wood Johnson Foundation *Anthology* series, examines this ambitious ten-state effort.

Wielawski explores why it is so difficult to recruit and retain health practitioners in rural settings and discusses other efforts—largely the federal government's National Health Service Corps—to encourage physicians and their families to move to rural areas. Focusing particularly on New Hampshire, Nebraska, and Virginia, Wielawski describes how the states participating in Practice Sights attempted to increase the availability of health care practitioners in rural areas.

Practice Sights was one of a number of Foundation programs—past and present—designed to improve health care services in rural areas. For example, the Foundation funded the Rural Infant Care program and the Rural Hospital Program of Extended-Care Services in the 1980s.[4] It currently supports the Southern Rural Access Program, which aims at increasing access to health care services in eight largely rural southern states.

---

1. Other chapters of the *To Improve Health and Health Care: The Robert Wood Johnson Foundation Anthology* series on the Foundation's work to increase access to health care are Isaacs, S. L., and Knickman, J. R. "Strategies for Improving Access to Health Care—Observations from The Robert Wood Johnson Foundation Anthology Series" (vol. V, 2002); Berk, M. L., and Schur, C. L. "A Review of the National Access-to-Care Surveys" (1997); and Holloway, M. Y. "Expanding Health Insurance for Children" (2000).

2. Other chapters of *The Robert Wood Johnson Foundation Anthology* series on the Foundation's workforce programs are Isaacs, S. L., Sandy, L. G., and Schroeder, S. A. "Improving the Health Care Workforce: Perspectives from Twenty-Four Years' Experience" (1997); and Keenan, T. "Support of Nurse-Practitioners and Physician Assistants" (1998–99).
3. Lois Bergeisen and Joel C. Cantor examine the Minority Medical Education Program in *To Improve Health and Health Care 2000: The Robert Wood Johnson Foundation Anthology.* San Francisco: Jossey-Bass, 2000.
4. Other chapters of *The Robert Wood Johnson Foundation Anthology* on the Foundation's rural health programs are Holloway, M. Y. "The Regionalized Perinatal Care Program" (2001); and Begley, S. "The Swing-Bed Program," Chapter Eleven in this volume.

—w— **D**avid Adams is a recent recruit to the health care system of Fairbury, Nebraska, population four thousand. An M.D., he works with four other family practitioners at the Fairbury Clinic, which is the source of primary care for most of Jefferson County—a large, rectangular chunk of farmland on the Nebraska-Kansas border. People travel an hour or more in all kinds of weather to get to the clinic, but they rarely complain of inconvenience. You don't have to go back many generations in rural America to hear firsthand what it was like when there was no doctor.

The inconveniences, moreover, are not borne entirely by patients. Adams and his colleagues must deliver twenty-first-century medicine in a setting that lacks the backup specialists and high-tech equipment they took for granted in training. The nearest specialists are in Beatrice, about fifty minutes from Fairbury. Lincoln, the state capital, where Adams trained, is more than a two-hour drive, and Omaha is three.

"We have to be able to do just about everything—the sore throat, the heart attack, the car wreck," says Adams, who happens to relish the challenge. Rural practitioners also speak of personal rewards that come through knowing their patients as fellow members of a community rather than as strangers passing through a busy urban practice.

Yet Adams and his sort are a scarce commodity. Only 2.6 percent of medical school graduates choose practice in a small town or rural area, according to the Association of American Medical Colleges. Over the years, this has resulted in a lopsided scenario in which fifty-one million rural Americans— roughly 20 percent of the nation's population—are being cared for by less than 10 percent of the nation's practicing physicians. Poor inner-city neighborhoods are similarly underserved because of a scarcity of health care providers.

This is not a new problem. The provider imbalance has worried academicians, government leaders, and health policy experts for more than thirty years. Periodically, efforts are launched to correct it, but there has been little measurable long-term improvement. Between 1980 and 1990, the number of federally designated Health Professional Shortage Areas, or HPSA, remained constant, at 1,956. The number of HPSAs steadily rose through the 1990s, despite an overall increase in the U.S. physician supply. By 2002, they totaled 3,168, of which 2,209 (70 percent) were in "nonmetropolitan" areas, as designated by the U.S. Health Resources and Services Administration. To eliminate these rural shortages would require successful recruitment and retention of 3,327 additional primary care physicians.[1]

There are several reasons for the continuing shortage. Income potential for a physician is lower in an underserved area, and many physicians today emerge from training with significant debt. Long hours, professional isolation, and lifestyle preferences are also cited as factors. Beyond these, however, rural health experts point to the absence of a national plan to improve the geographic distribution of health care providers. Efforts to date have been largely piecemeal, with little coordination among government and private sector initiatives.

Perhaps the best known of these initiatives is the National Health Service Corps, made up of physicians who agree to be posted to underserved areas of the United States in exchange for repayment of medical education loans. The Corps has been an excellent source of physicians for localities that would have had a hard time recruiting on their own. Unfortunately, Corps physicians tend to leave when their contracts are up, sending these communities scurrying once again for what is still the most essential component of any health care system: a doctor.

Historically, states have not, until recently, paid much attention to their medically underserved areas, often considering them a federal responsibility, similar to the provision of health insurance (Medicaid and Medicare), welfare, or housing support for the very poor. Some states have experimented with home-grown solutions, such as loan repayment and *locum tenens* (substitute doctor) programs, to ease the economic and workload burden on providers. The majority, however, simply clamored for more National Health Service Corps doctors, more federally funded clinics for poor and uninsured patients, more federal response in general.

Finger-pointing at the feds may be convenient for governors, but it didn't sit well with state public health professionals. Just as poverty and a lack of insurance have measurable consequences for the health of individuals, so does a medically underserved area have consequences for population health. Population health is the means by which public health professionals measure their own performance. As the provider shortages persisted, it became apparent that medically underserved areas were dragging down population health statistics. People in these communities *are* sicker than residents of communities with sufficient doctors and health centers.[2] They also tend to have a lower immunization rate, higher infant mortality, and other measurable deficits. Smart program design, compelling health promotion campaigns, determined outreach workers—all fail without health care providers to deliver the goods.

It was against this backdrop that The Robert Wood Johnson Foundation decided to offer a challenge to states to come up with more comprehensive approaches to recruitment and retention of rural and inner-city health care providers. The $16.5 million program was called Practice Sights: State Primary Care Development Strategies. Its overriding goal was to improve access to primary health care by increasing the number of providers in underserved areas. Physicians were only one type of provider envisioned by those designing Practice Sights. The program also sought to introduce physicians' assistants, nurse practitioners, and nurse midwives into underserved communities, and to improve the regulatory climate in states that restricted these mid-level practitioners from fully using their skills.

Success in landing recruits is only half the task; the other half is, How do you get them to stay? The Foundation had more ambitious goals than to merely duplicate underserved communities' experience with the National Health Service Corps. To this end, Practice Sights challenged states to come up with ways to make medical practice in these communities economically viable and to ameliorate the conditions that lead health care providers to leave, among them professional isolation and excessive workload.

Practice Sights was authorized by the Foundation in the fall of 1991 and ran through 1998. A National Program Office, or NPO, was established at the North Carolina Foundation for Alternative Health, under the direction of James D. Bernstein. Practice Sights clearly struck a chord with state health officials eager to emancipate themselves from dependence on disparate federal programs: forty-four of the fifty states responded to the NPO's request for proposals. Of these, fifteen were successful in winning Practice Sights planning grants of up to $100,000.

The planning grant was to be used to lay the groundwork for effective recruiting and retention of physicians and midlevel practitioners. Planning activities included assembling interagency working groups; building liaison between state entities and underserved communities; developing statewide information systems to track vacancies and advertise for candidates; and removing licensing or other barriers to effective use of physician assistants, nurse practitioners, and other non-M.D. primary care providers.

Practice Sights moved into its second phase, implementation, in the summer of 1994. The Foundation authorized a new round of grants averaging $800,000 that states could use over three years to carry out ideas honed in the planning phase. Of the fifteen states that received planning grants, ten were successful in winning implementation grants: Idaho, Kentucky, Minnesota, Nebraska, New Hampshire, New Mexico, New York, Pennsylvania, South Dakota, and Virginia. These states mostly focused on underserved rural areas, even though Practice Sights originally aimed at addressing human resource shortages in both rural and inner-city settings. As a result, the collective Practice Sights effort emphasized rural issues.

—w— Program Overview

Practice Sights swam against the economic and cultural tide of American medicine and long-established trends among medical school graduates to head for metropolitan practices, where pay and prestige are greatest. The program set three goals for grantees:

1. To increase the number of primary care providers in underserved areas
2. To improve reimbursement levels and working conditions in underserved areas so they have a better chance of attracting and keeping providers
3. To increase the state's capacity to support primary care systems

For a single site to achieve even one of these goals in the relatively short run of the program would have been impressive. To make headway during the particular years of Practice Sights is nothing short of amazing, for there has probably been no period of greater upheaval in the history of the American health care system.

Practice Sights' debut coincided with widespread public and political concern about the plight of the medically uninsured and the unreliability of the private insurance system. Passage of some type of national health reform was considered imminent. The universal health coverage included in most proposals before Congress was especially important in the context of Practice Sights, since medically underserved areas have a relatively high proportion of uninsured or inadequately insured patients. If federal reform gave these patients a means to pay for medical treatment, health systems and providers in underserved areas would benefit as well. This could only enhance the prospects for successful recruiting and retention. No one designing Practice Sights in the early 1990s or applying for one of its grants could have anticipated the failure of President Bill Clinton's Health Security Plan in 1994, and the domino effect on all other reform proposals. The timing was particularly onerous; congressional leaders declared health reform dead only a month after Practice Sights' most adventuresome states entered the high-risk implementation phase.

There followed a dizzying period of health care system reorganization and consolidation, in anticipation of a managed care juggernaut. Rural health systems were caught up in the general frenzy. New Hampshire, for one, saw its rural hospitals scrambling to buy out physician practices, or to affiliate with neighboring hospitals. These local health systems believed their best defense against the shrewd deal making of gigantic multistate managed care companies was to array patients and other assets into a unified front. The feared alternative was to be picked off one by one and lowballed on reimbursement rates. These turned out to be costly strategies, fueled by fear. By the late 1990s, it was clear that managed care companies had little interest in rural markets. But Practice Sights was already well along by then.

"There were pluses and minuses to that period," says Jonathan Stewart, director of the Community Health Institute in Concord, New Hampshire, a collaborator on that state's Practice Sights project. Pluses included an unusual receptivity to new ideas among normally tradition-bound rural physicians and hospitals. On the other hand, with day-to-day survival a foremost concern, it was difficult to get people focused on long-term systemic improvements.

Another wild card in Practice Sights was the character of rural medicine in each of the participating states. It is a running joke among rural providers that the only people who can comfortably generalize about their working conditions are researchers studying them from the climate-controlled comfort of an urban think tank. That said, rural providers themselves tend to generalize from their own experience, which may not be the norm for others. The Practice Sights states exemplified this variation in functional definitions of *rural* and *medically needy*. New Hampshire, for example, has a hospital every thirty miles or so in its underserved North Country. Providers and patients in larger states such as South Dakota and Nebraska would consider this pure luxury (that is, until they tried driving New Hampshire's twisty North Country roads in January). As for the needs of Virginia's rural communities, well, it depends upon which part of the state you're talking about. Says Deborah D. Oswalt, executive director of the Virginia Health Care Foundation and a Practice Sights collaborator:

> Our southwest tail—that's Appalachia—has such difficult terrain that it can take you an hour to go ten miles, especially if you get behind a coal truck. We've got Southside Virginia, which is a very different place with very different people. It is still very agricultural. More than a third of the population over age twenty-five in Southside has not completed high school. There is still housing in some places with dirt floors and no indoor plumbing. Then we have the Northern Neck, which is in eastern Virginia near Chesapeake Bay. We have a lot of watermen there who make their living by fishing and crabbing and oystering, and their health issues and travel issues are very different from those of the mountain and Southside people. You simply cannot generalize about rural health needs, not even in a single state.

Practice Sights had a final twist. In addition to traditional grant funding, the Foundation offered participating states a highly atypical business deal. Essentially, the Foundation took on the role of a bank, sending seed money to grantees so that they in turn could create a loan fund to give rural providers access to low-interest capital. The Foundation loans—called Program-Related Investments, or PRIs—ranged from $700,000 to $1.5 million.[3] Payback with interest was required within ten years. Only four of the ten Practice Sights grantees took the PRI option, and it proved to be a rocky experiment for all concerned, with mixed results.

—ᴍᴍ— A Showcase of Lessons from Three States

The lessons of Practice Sights found their best showcases in three states: New Hampshire, Nebraska, and Virginia. These states exemplify the rural diversity that characterized the program, and their experiences underscore the importance of local fine-tuning if a national workforce strategy ever materializes. These states also emerged as unusually illustrative of how the Practice Sights program played out. New Hampshire used Practice Sights to build a strong statewide provider recruitment system, but it did not develop a loan program and had limited success in other areas of the project, such as improved working conditions. Nebraska's greatest accomplishments came in organizing balkanized rural providers into mutually supportive hospital and physician networks, thereby reducing professional isolation and improving economic stability. But its PRI loan program was a colossal failure. Virginia made little progress in moving recruiting to the state level; the rural physician workforce continues to be replenished through direct recruiting by local practices. However, the Virginia project took a $700,000 seed loan from the Foundation and leveraged it into a successful revolving fund that to date has issued nearly $6 million in low-interest financing for health-related investments in underserved communities.

Recruiting

Why would your average debt-laden medical school graduate choose to work in a setting with limited income potential, long hours, and gravely compromised social options? This was the challenge to Practice Sights leaders. In New Hampshire, the sales job belongs to Stephanie Pagliuca.

Pagliuca is program manager of the New Hampshire Recruitment Center. Located in Concord, the state capital, the Recruitment Center is a not-for-profit enterprise created through Practice Sights. Its track record is impressive. By the end of 2001, the state had filled just about every vacancy in its medically underserved areas, including the North Country, a sparsely populated region that borders Canada. Overall, since the inception of Practice Sights, a total of 131 physicians and nurse practitioners have been successfully recruited in New

Hampshire. Twenty-six percent of those recruited went to HPSAs, a federal designation for regions where the ratio of patients to physicians is greater than 3,500:1. Twenty-nine percent went to Medically Underserved Areas, so-called because population and health demographics—including age, poverty, and a high rate of low-birth-weight babies—show a need for more doctors. The remaining 45 percent went to practices elsewhere in the state.

The Recruitment Center was part of a broad Practice Sights–fueled effort to address a patchwork health care infrastructure in New Hampshire, especially in its North Country. Population and the lion's share of health care professionals and facilities were concentrated in the southern half of the state. Public health workers were scattered and poorly coordinated. The state used the umbrella of Practice Sights to join forces with local community health care organizations. Besides the Recruitment Center, New Hampshire's Practice Sights leaders created the Community Health Institute, which provided consulting services to medically needy communities, administered a state loan repayment fund to enhance recruiting of health care providers with sizeable school debt, and developed preceptor programs with local colleges and universities, through which medical and nursing students were placed in underserved areas. The Institute, in collaboration with the state health department, gained new federal support for New Hampshire by qualifying communities for community health center grants.

The standout legacy of Practice Sights in New Hampshire, however, is the Recruitment Center. Initially supported by Practice Sights grant money and state contributions, the Recruitment Center today is largely self-sustaining. It operates on a fee-for-service basis, charging hospitals, clinics, and physician practices about half what they would pay for commercial recruiting assistance.

Ironically, one of New Hampshire's strongest assets is the relative weakness of what Practice Sights architects thought would be the program's anchor: state health departments. New Hampshire's history is one of decentralized government; its state agencies are bare-bones, and the electorate consistently votes against anything that would expand the power of state government over local community rule.

"The basic social and decision-making unit in New Hampshire is the town—the community," says James W. Squires, a surgeon and former state senator. He currently heads the Endowment for Health, a foundation working to improve health care access in New Hampshire. "It is not the county; it is not a hospital cachement area; it is not a demographic unit; and it is certainly not state government. Every town has its own police force; every one has its own ambulance, fire department, and education system."

A single town is not the ideal unit for advancing statewide improvements in health systems or workforce, but state officials in New Hampshire are used to modest stature and are adept at getting around the handicap.

"We know right off that we will never have the expertise in state government to guide each community to fulfill its health care needs," says John Bonds, a state health services planner and a Practice Sights project director. "So we are very good at creating community and statewide coalitions to help formulate and carry out programs. Everything is done under contract to existing community-based agencies: visiting nurses, home health care agencies, and the rest."

As a result, Practice Sights in New Hampshire spent almost no time bottled up in health department bureaucracy; instead it immediately began to work with mostly private sector coalitions with established credibility in the health care community. (By contrast, Nebraska's project lacked staff for more than two years because of a statewide hiring freeze that barred health officials from filling the grant-funded position.) Bonds, Pagliuca, and other Practice Sights leaders were able to turn to these community-based coalitions for ideas and practical assistance in implementing the goals of Practice Sights.

For example, at the outset of the 1990s, New Hampshire had only one federally funded community health center, even though numerous localities met the criteria to qualify for federal assistance. What they lacked was the leadership necessary to mount a successful application. This was the genesis of the New Hampshire Practice Sights' consulting arm, the Community Health Institute. State and private sector health leaders saw an opportunity to mobilize communities under the aegis of Practice Sights, since new health centers with funded staff positions for underserved communities would be consistent with the program's goals. The applications were carefully timed to prevent one New Hampshire community from knocking another out of contention. The collaborative approach resulted in nine new health centers—a significant accomplishment for a small state in a competitive federal program.

In building the recruitment center's capacity, Pagliuca and her colleagues took a similarly collaborative approach. She recalls:

> We started out simply responding to requests for candidates to fill vacancies. We did some educating of practices to think about using nurse practitioners, because the University of New Hampshire had an emerging training program. Then we started to link up with other organizations in New Hampshire that were getting similar calls: the medical society, the hospital association. Then we got the nurse practitioner and physician assistant societies joining. Then we linked up to our state loan repayment program, and strengthened our relationship with the National Health Service Corps. That gave us a more comprehensive package to offer candidates.
>
> We also helped create marketing materials for the practices, advertisements for publications read by physicians such as *The New England Journal of Medicine, Family Physician Recruiter* newsletter, *OBG Management*, and so on.

Gavin Muir was one of the recruiting successes. Muir graduated from Temple University's medical school in 1995 and trained in family practice in a Pueblo, Colorado, residency program strongly oriented to rural practice. He began talking to Pagliuca about job possibilities in August 1997, which was eleven months before he completed training.

"I had some very specific requirements and after that I was flexible," Muir says. "Number one, I wanted to work some place where I could practice obstetrics because I put so much blood, sweat, and tears into the advanced obstetrics program in Pueblo. Number two, I wanted some place that would help me with my loans. I had $160,000 in medical school debt. Number three, my wife and I wanted to be reasonably close to our families—she's from Buffalo. Number four, I wanted a decent quality of life."

All of these criteria were met by the Manchester Community Health Center, where Muir is currently medical director. The health center is one of New Hampshire's new ones, located in a rare pocket of urban need. A manufacturing city of about one hundred thousand residents, Manchester is home to a large immigrant community, with a recent influx of Bosnian and Sudanese refugees. Muir is delighted with his job for professional, practical, and personal reasons.

"I work a four-day week," he says, which enables him to spend time with his wife and four-year-old daughter. "I'm in the fourth year of federal loan repayment because I work in a federally designated underserved area. This means $120,000 in loans paid off so far by the feds. I love what I am doing; I enjoy living where I am. All my friends who did National Health Service Corps got out as soon as they could because their spouses were ready to kill them. But this is a place where people would love to live. An hour from the beach, an hour from the mountains, a couple of hours from Boston."

Pagliuca acknowledges recruiting advantages for New Hampshire in the state's natural beauty and its relative proximity to a major city like Boston. The Recruiting Center's Website emphasizes these attributes on each informational screen, with luscious photographs of lakes, mountains, and majestic forests. Of course, the appeal is not universal.

Pagliuca recalls a deluge of job seekers from 1996 to 1997, all foreign-born and looking to bypass immigration requirements that they return to their own country after training. A loophole was the J-1 visa program, which exempted foreign physicians working in medically underserved areas of the United States. Pagliuca's experience with one of these physicians illustrates another recruiting responsibility: screening out an unqualified applicant or, simply, a poor fit. As she recalls:

> Many of them I could barely understand over the phone, their English was so poor. How could they practice in our rural areas? We were recruiting for retention, and the lack of cultural outlets for these physicians really didn't make it realistic. There were no appropriate places of worship, no ethnic food stores, that sort of thing.
>
> I had one physician from a Middle Eastern country who was interested in a position in our North Country. But he was a vegetarian. There is a real problem getting fresh produce up there in winter. That's a genuine concern, although a lot of times the physicians don't really think about these things. It is our job to bring up these lifestyle and cultural issues with every candidate. Think about this: "You are going to a rural town. What does that mean in terms of social outlets? Does your spouse want to work? Are there opportunities there?"
>
> Initially, I felt a little uncomfortable asking these questions about spouses, or dealing with issues of same-sex couples or racial and cultural issues. How many of these questions are discriminatory? We worry about this, but then we realize

that the physicians are just as interested in going to a community that will be a good fit for them. We do an awful lot of handholding on both sides.

In the case of the Middle Eastern physician, a site visit helped clarify realities for all concerned. What Pagliuca could not convey during the office interview was amply demonstrated during the visit, which included a stop at the local grocery store. The physician was dismayed by the skimpy produce section, which his family would depend upon to uphold cultural and religious dietary practices. In subsequent interviews with local physicians and hospital officials, he brought this up as a concern. Eager for help with the patient load, the physicians assured him that he and his family would soon love meat. They even offered to supply his wife with recipes and take him on moose hunting trips.

"He came back to Concord and withdrew his application," Pagliuca recalls. "He told me, 'I am not going to change my beliefs and practices just for a job.' It was a satisfactory conclusion. It wasn't going to be a good fit for anyone."

In Nebraska and Virginia, recruiting continues to be a function of local practices, although Practice Sights did help to establish statewide databanks cataloguing the characteristics of locales, provider needs, and other considerations. Unlike New Hampshire, which is a relatively small state, Nebraska and Virginia must contend with significant distance and diversity in their health systems. The experience of Practice Sights leaders there suggests that a regional approach to recruiting might work better in a larger state, or even that several states with common geography and demographics might collaborate in recruiting. In Nebraska, for example, practices like the one David Adams joined in Fairbury are the easiest to recruit for because the community has a full-service local hospital, urban centers are relatively close, and the Fairbury practice has enough doctors for collegiality and a reasonable work schedule. It is more difficult to sell physicians on a remote community such as Benkelman, six hours' drive from Lincoln, or Calloway, where the district hospital's medical staff consists of a single doctor—a 24/7 job if there ever was one. "I wouldn't say Benkelman is exactly the end of the world," says Dennis Berens of Nebraska's Office of Rural Health. "But you can see it from there."

Even to recruit someone who is as ideal on paper as David Adams was takes creativity. The body of research on rural physicians suggests that those who work out best grow up in a small town; marry someone from a small town; and have a self-confident, take-charge personality. David Adams is all of these. But he brought requirements to the table that typify expectations of the newest medical school graduates—a reality for rural recruiting no less than for a large group practice. His negotiations with the Fairbury Clinic underscore the personal and highly individualized dynamic that Stephanie Pagliuca has found essential to success in New Hampshire.

Adams didn't want to work the twelve-hour days that his seniors in the Fairbury practice considered routine, and he was equally tough-minded about night and weekend duty. He wanted an income sufficient to meet lifestyle and financial goals. Indeed, most states are finding they cannot recruit rural physicians without a guaranteed first-year income of $100,000 to $125,000. And though it's true that Adams has a spouse to help in his transition to small-town America, that's not *her* complete job description, as it might have been a generation ago. Mrs. David Adams also happens to be a physician. Any practice hoping to recruit David Adams, M.D., had to come up with an equally appealing position for Kari Adams, M.D. The physician partners in the Fairbury Clinic decided it was worth it to go up to five doctors from four to accommodate both Adamses.

Virginia's rural areas are experimenting with private recruiting on a larger scale. In its southwestern Appalachia region, the not-for-profit Carilion Medical Group handles recruiting for forty-four affiliated private practices. The group has 175 physician members and is a subsidiary of the Carilion Health System, the largest hospital network in western Virginia. The health system provides income subsidies for new physician recruits and for members of the medical group working in extreme poverty areas. For its part, the medical group runs educational workshops and has linked the practices to computerized information systems to keep its members up to date on the latest developments in medical science.

This last element is critical, says James G. Nuckolls, a rural physician in Galax, who is the group's medical director. He emphasizes what so often is left out of the numbers discussion dominating conventional thinking on rural recruitment: rural populations need *good* doctors, not just warm bodies.

"We do our best to recruit the people that seem to be good, but then we watch them real close during the first year," Nuckolls says. "We want to make sure they are real doctors, not just playing at being a doctor to fulfill lifestyle needs. It's like that saying: 'He ain't no cowboy till you seen him ride.' We support them every way we can, but we've got to see that they are hard workers and team players."

Landing quality recruits, however, is only the first step. Keeping them sharp is as much a part of the retention formula as income and lifestyle support, according to Nuckolls. "The thing that happens to rural doctors is that they get isolated and can no longer measure the true quality of their work," he says. "They start to measure themselves by the compliments they receive from patients. Pretty soon, the doctor's head gets so swelled that he's a walking deity. The fact is, medical quality is best judged by one's peers. You've got to be in contact with peers, challenged on the science and so forth, to keep yourself sharp and interested."

Improving Economic Conditions

The dream of Nebraska's rural health planners is to have a dozen networks scattered about the state, mimicking the Carilion system in southwest Virginia. But with Practice Sights they were starting from scratch, and with two strikes against them. First, the historic evolution of the state's rural health system had left individual hospitals and physicians unusually isolated from one another, compared with smaller and more populous states. Second, many of them were struggling financially at the launch of Practice Sights and had little capital to invest in systems change.

Nebraska is very rural. Its two urban centers, Lincoln and Omaha, are on the eastern edge, about an hour apart. These cities are also the center of tertiary care medicine and medical education. As you head west toward the Panhandle region, bordering Wyoming, towns become smaller and farther apart. Large sections of the state don't even qualify as rural, falling instead into the public health definition of *frontier*. No statewide entity—no health department, hospital association, or medical society—can generalize about the characteristics and needs of Nebraska's rural health systems. They pretty much operate as a collection of local fiefdoms, some good, some less so, all fiercely independent in character. This defining ethos goes back to pioneer times, when an isolated community had to develop self-sufficiency or perish. It continues today for remarkably similar reasons. Of 534 incorporated communities in Nebraska, 90 percent have fewer than twenty-five hundred people. But with an area of 77,355 square miles, Nebraska is more than eight times the size of New Hampshire. The one-on-one handholding that Stephanie Pagliuca can do from Concord is not possible from Lincoln. Just to sit down with physicians in the Panhandle means an eight-hour drive.

"You do not come in as a state person in Nebraska and say, 'This is how it is going to be,'" says David Palm of the state Department of Health and Human Services, who led the Practice Sights project in Nebraska and has folded his lanky 6' 6" frame into state cars for many such trips. "You have to soft-pedal everything, and be very respectful of how the communities have traditionally done things, and think carefully about what we at the state level can do to help them accomplish *their* goals."

Dennis Berens, who heads Nebraska's Office of Rural Health and was the mild-mannered Palm's colleague on Practice Sights, adds, "People here don't like outsiders coming in and telling them what to do—not from Lincoln, not from Washington, and not from some big foundation in Princeton. If we tried to do that, it would be 'Just put the money in a bag and leave it at the outskirts of town. . . .'"

Nebraska's health officials used the Practice Sights grant to organize the state's diverse and far-flung regions into five provider networks. With varying degrees of success, the networks worked collaboratively to recruit additional health care providers and to provide educational forums for members—both goals of Practice Sights. The networks also joined forces with the University of Nebraska and various state agencies to expand scholarship, loan repayment, and *locum tenens* programs for health care providers willing to work in an underserved area. Practice Sights leaders were also successful in spurring legislative action to eliminate certain practice restrictions on physicians' assistants so they could help alleviate the provider shortage.

As in New Hampshire, Nebraska's Practice Sights leaders got unexpected momentum from rural providers' panic over managed care, which spurred interest in collaborative action. In southeast Nebraska, physicians had already formed the Southeast Rural Physicians Alliance to negotiate managed care contracts and explore other business-oriented group activities such as bulk purchasing of supplies and better rates for malpractice insurance. Similarly, the hospitals in that region had formed the Blue River Valley Hospital Network. Seeing an opportunity for fully integrating the health care delivery system, Palm suggested that the organizations take the next step of collaborating with one another. This led to formation of the Rural Comprehensive Care Network, a physician and hospital alliance made up of local health systems in seventeen counties in Nebraska's southeastern corner.

The southeast network—which today remains the strongest of those organized under Practice Sights—undertakes a variety of projects for its members, including negotiating lower-cost bulk purchase of supplies and better rates on malpractice insurance. It has also started some medical quality-improvement projects. But there is no mistaking the driving force behind these activities: the economic survival of local hospitals and physicians. Even the medical quality-improvement projects are oriented to the bottom line; one purpose is to prove to local residents that they needn't drive all the way to Lincoln for first-rate primary medical care.

Palm, Berens, and other Practice Sights leaders sought to sell the program's goals—improved recruiting, better use of midlevel practitioners, and so on—in the context of these overtly financial concerns. Indeed, Practice Sights stripped down was very much about economic survival. At some point in the program's five-year course, every grantee realized the need to meld principle—improving health care access for rural populations—with the practical: ensuring the financial viability of rural physicians and hospitals. In Nebraska, however, cold reality was a companion from Day One. Consider:

- Pushed to explore the possibility of expanding the capacity of his solo practice with a nurse practitioner, an older rural physician was shocked to discover that the going rate for a salary—about $60,000 a year—exceeded his own income. He gave up, unable to imagine how to fund the position, given the general poverty of his community.

- In the Panhandle, where state health officials hoped to stimulate formation of a rural health coalition similar to the one in southeast Nebraska, nine of the region's thirteen hospital administrators turned over in two years, a leadership instability related to the very conditions Practice Sights sought to alleviate for physicians.

■ Reimbursement rates set by Medicare, the dominant payer in rural Nebraska, were among the worst in the country because of historically low fees charged by physicians and hospitals.

"We had older physicians who were still charging five, eight, and ten dollars a visit," Palm says. "That was going to be a real problem if managed care came in and tried to negotiate on the basis of that rate. We realized we needed to lay some building blocks for improving recruiting and many other aspects of rural health in Nebraska. You can't look just at recruitment and retention as a single issue. The solutions really have to be multifaceted, and you can't attribute them to one program or one set of goals."

Just about everything Nebraska experimented with under Practice Sights came down to money—mostly the lack of it. In its effort to lay building blocks, the health department, as Practice Sights' lead agency, brought in a variety of partners, including the Nebraska Economic Development Corporation, the medical school at the University of Nebraska, the Office of Rural Health, and even private community entities such as the Saint Elizabeth's Foundation. The latter was asked to develop a *locum tenens* program, through which medical residents and emergency room or retired physicians in Lincoln and Omaha would cover for rural physicians who needed a break. Surveys of doctors and potential recruits showed enthusiasm for such a program, but Nebraska's rural health systems could pay only twenty to thirty dollars an hour, which was about fifteen dollars under market. Moonlighters could earn more—and conveniently—by filling openings in the cities or suburbs. "Fifty miles was about the limit of what they wanted to travel," says Donna K. Hammack, of the Saint Elizabeth's Foundation. "Our rural areas were a lot farther than that."

The failure of the experiment convinced Practice Sights leaders of the necessity of locally based human resource solutions. But human resources could not be bolstered without significant improvement in rural health's bottom line—exactly the focus of the program's constituents. Practice Sights leaders redirected their efforts from the specific goals articulated by the grant program to Palm's building blocks. Specifically, they set out to help rural hospitals take advantage of federal programs—designation as a Critical Access Hospital or

Rural Health Clinic—that would vastly improve the revenue stream for providers. Both programs afford an opportunity for qualified providers to secure higher reimbursement under Medicare and Medicaid.

The strategy had remarkable success, similar to New Hampshire's with gaining federally funded health centers. The number of physician practices earning Rural Health Clinic status went from five to seventy-seven in Nebraska; the number of Critical Access Hospitals went from zero to fifty-five, largely as a result of the momentum gained from Practice Sights.

Other building blocks include the startup of three additional hospital/physician networks modeled on southeast Nebraska's Rural Comprehensive Care Network. Practice Sights leaders also gave support to University of Nebraska efforts aimed at creating a supply of health professionals. As it is, the majority of physicians practicing in Nebraska are graduates of the University of Nebraska or its medical school. But to build a supply of *rural* physicians, the university's medical center now sponsors an eighth grade science fair to identify talented students in rural areas. These youngsters become eligible for scholarships to state colleges and, if successful there, are guaranteed admission to a health profession graduate program at the University, including medicine, pharmacy, dentistry, physical therapy, and occupational therapy. The medical school has a special Rural Health Opportunities Program, which rotates students through rural practices to give them hands-on experience. An added benefit is courtesy faculty status for the students' physician mentors, giving these relatively isolated practitioners a connection to the university.

The Loan Program

Virginia was one of only four Practice Sights grantees that dared to tango with The Robert Wood Johnson Foundation's Program-Related Investment idea. The Virginia project was ultimately successful, but only after protracted and dizzying negotiations that left other Practice Sights grantees badly winded. Nebraska had the worst experience and ended up returning the Foundation's money.

The PRI was a relatively new undertaking for the Foundation when program officers made it part of Practice Sights, though conceptually it had been a recognized vehicle for charitable funding since the Tax Reform Act of 1969. Instead of a grant, the Foundation proposed to *lend* seed money to Practice Sights grantees for a revolving loan fund that would give health care providers access to capital at a favorable interest rate. Unlike a grant, whose use is restricted to project personnel and operating costs, a loan fund could legitimately finance bricks-and-mortar-type investment consistent with program goals. In Practice Sights, one could imagine many such uses, from upgrading a rural physician's office equipment to rehabilitating a Main Street storefront for use as a primary care clinic. The Foundation expected grantees to round up local partners to match the seed loan, five to one. It also required payback of the Foundation's loan plus 3 percent interest within ten years.

The loan arrangement was the problem. It saddled Practice Sights grantees with an unusual and intimidating management task. Most of their experience was with grants, which, once you land them, can be freely spent for defined purposes. About the only way you can get into trouble is if you take a Hawaiian vacation or otherwise abuse a funder's trust. The essence of successful grant management is prudence and integrity. Practice Sights leaders were confident that they could manage the grants part of the program.

The PRI requirements, however, challenged their financial acumen, of which they were less confident. Among several noteworthy consequences was unusual timidity in this area of Practice Sights. The grantees stuck the loan money in bank certificates of deposit, the most conservative form of investment. Their primary concern was safeguarding the Foundation's money and earning the required interest before even a penny went out into the field. In this, the PRI experiment contrasted sharply with The Robert Wood Johnson Foundation's long-avowed mission of stimulating innovation and risk taking in the field, which unquestionably occurred in Practice Sights grant-funded areas.

Peter Goodwin, the Foundation's vice president for finance, acknowledges conceptual miscalculations with the PRI. "It was a new business for us, and at the time we weren't very good at it," he says. Among other things, Foundation staff members did not think through the operational difficulties conferred by the loan repayment conditions. The staff members thought the loan would be educational for grantees, stimulating greater financial sophistication than a grant could about how to use money to greatest effect. But neither the Foundation nor the grantees joining in this experiment realized the complexity of the world they were entering. Fluctuating interest rates during Practice Sights' tenure were only one problem. There was also the surprising naïveté of the loan program's intended beneficiaries: rural health care providers. The PRI experience was instructive for the Foundation and grantees alike, but its structural complexity interfered with program goals.

In Nebraska's case, it utterly defeated them. "We probably spent eight or nine months negotiating the terms with Robert Wood Johnson, the legal and finance people," recalls George Frye, executive vice president of the Nebraska Economic Development Corporation, or NEDCO, which handled the rollout of the loan fund. By the time agreement was reached, in December 1996, interest rates had dropped too low for NEDCO to offer a competitive rate and still make the money necessary to pay back the Foundation. Moreover, Nebraska found that it needed to sell the idea of borrowing to rural providers and then walk them through the loan process. They needed much more help than NEDCO's usual business customers did.

"We basically were trying to do this in a place as big as Nebraska with the existing NEDCO staff, which is pretty small," Frye said. "It's me, and I'm part-time, one full-time loan packager, and one portfolio manager. There was no money for marketing or extra staff. If we could have just had one person dedicated to going around and acquainting people with this program, I think we could have done better."

In the end, Nebraska's Community Primary Care Loan Program made only two loans. The first one ended in default; the second one financed a bailout of the first one. At that point, Practice Sights leaders concluded that the experiment was too high-risk, especially with only a ten-year loan cycle. They retrenched to priority number one: paying back the Foundation. In December 2000, their investments succeeded in restoring the full loan amount plus 3 percent. Nebraska promptly cut a check to the Foundation and withdrew from the experiment.

Virginia encountered many of the same structural problems but overcame them. The loan program established under Practice Sights, called the Healthy Communities Loan Fund, continues to grow in volume and scope. It is run under the auspices of a private philanthropy, the Virginia Health Care

Foundation, which was a collaborator with the Virginia Department of Health in Practice Sights. The fund surpassed the $4 million mark in late 2001 and recently extended eligibility for a loan to mental health professionals and pharmacists. Ironically, at $700,000, Virginia's seed loan was the smallest in the program. Nebraska, by contrast, got $1.5 million.

Why was Virginia's experience so different from Nebraska's? Deborah D. Oswalt, of the Virginia Health Care Foundation, has a quick answer: "We had real bankers with commercial lending experience helping us every step of the way." Getting "real bankers" on board was an idea forged by Oswalt's concern over the PRI's complexity, which also raised eyebrows on her governing board.

"The fact that it was a loan and that we had to repay it and pay interest and so on definitely influenced how we handled the $700,000," Oswalt says. "It is not as if we were some banking gurus. We're a nonprofit foundation. What did we know about any of that sophisticated high-finance stuff? My board wanted to be sure I wasn't sitting there making loan decisions. This helped us develop a real working partnership with the banking community."

Oswalt and her staff came up with an ingenious method of identifying the best bank for their purposes. They superimposed a map of Virginia's underserved areas on the branch networks of Virginia-based banks and found that First Virginia Banks had 310 branches in Virginia, many of them in the areas Practice Sights deemed eligible for lending. Says Oswalt:

> I can't overemphasize the importance of the relationship with the bank to our success. We learned so much from them and got help in ways we never expected. When we ran into declining interest rates, we actually questioned whether we should continue. It was getting impossible to offer the favorable loan terms we wanted: prime rate, no points, no prepayment penalties to make this a really good deal for our rural providers. But the bank was able to come through with special package deals like free checking and all those other extras banks offer good customers. So, yes, maybe the doctors could go elsewhere and get a better rate, but they wouldn't get the individual attention and help they get from us.

The bank also prints and mails the health care foundation's informational brochures, subsidizes other marketing costs, and works closely with Lilia Mayer, the Healthy Communities Loan Fund's indispensable point person. As in Nebraska, Virginia found that it needed a dedicated staff person to promote the project and respond to inquiries. The expertise that they assumed highly educated people such as doctors would bring to the transaction simply wasn't there.

"We learned to our surprise that some physicians are poor businessmen," Oswalt says. "Their bookkeeping was very rudimentary. They just wanted to treat patients, and they really did not know how to assess their assets or how much of a loan they could handle or how to develop a business plan. So Lilia began to incorporate the literature of the Small Business Administration in our mailings to help them out. It was never envisioned that we would be a technical assistance program in addition to a loan program, but that is how it turned out."

First Virginia Banks has reaped rewards as well. Tentative at first, the bank has steadily ramped up its support, recognizing the loan program's benefit to core business. First Virginia competes with larger banks by cultivating grassroots customers as opposed to major national corporations, according to John P. Salop, a senior vice president and liaison to the Healthy Communities Loan Fund. The bank recently received the American Bankers Association's ACTION Award in recognition of its Practice Sights contributions. Still, Salop admits to some early qualms.

"This was new, it was different, so, sure, there were people at the bank with reservations," he says. "The biggest fear was that you would be spinning your wheels, that it would never get going because the underpinnings were weak. You don't want to waste your time. We said we would be willing to accept less"—in the way of interest and collateral, for instance—"but they still had to be profitable loans if this was going to be a long-term thing. Everything has to make economic sense."

With the experience of Practice Sights as a guide, The Robert Wood Johnson Foundation took another look at the economic sense of requiring loan repayment plus interest. Specifically, in the case of Virginia's Healthy Communities Loan Fund, the Foundation decided in early 2002 to forgive the 3 percent interest requirement entirely. Bank interest rates had dropped so precipitously during 2001 that the loan fund barely earned enough to cover program operating costs, never mind the Foundation's fee. Recognizing this difficulty, the Foundation essentially converted the terms of the PRI agreement to those of an interest-free loan.

Current Foundation programs are experimenting with PRIs whose seed money comes in the form of grants, not loans. The term of the grant may also be indefinitely extended, eliminating the inflexibility of a short loan cycle.

—⚭— Conclusions

Practice Sights aimed at improving health care by easing conditions that discourage health care providers from working in underserved rural or inner city settings. The program also sought to build capacity at the state level to address workforce issues, thus reducing states' dependence upon federal initiatives.

Collectively, grantees succeeded in recruiting 867 health care providers; the total includes physicians, nurse midwives, nurse practitioners, and physician assistants. New Hampshire had a net increase in physicians. Nebraska, by contrast, finished the project with exactly the same number of rural physicians as when Practice Sights started. But the state's success in shoring up the financial underpinnings of rural health systems via Critical Access Hospital and Rural Health Clinic designations resulted in hiring a significant number of midlevel providers, where before there had been none.

To the numerical scorecard, Practice Sights added valuable insights into the alchemy of successful recruiting and retention of health care providers. Notably, it illustrated the links between the rural health care workforce and larger economic, political, and workforce trends in the United States. If a local hospital is too cash-strapped to hire a midlevel health professional to help with night and weekend emergency room coverage, there isn't much hope for improving the physician's call schedule. Similarly, a revolving door of providers and administrators bodes ill for any health system's ability to meet community needs. As Nebraska's David Palm observed, no single program or initiative can tackle all of the factors that discourage providers from working in certain areas. But Practice Sights shed new light on the dimensions of the problem and challenged conventional thinking in some areas.

The connection between health care and the larger environment plays out daily in recruiting. Success depends upon nimbly tailoring a pitch to current market demands. However, recruiters seasoned by Practice Sights learned to take the stated expectations of today's medical school graduates with more of a grain of salt than health systems researchers or senior physicians seem to. This last group is uniformly exasperated by recent candidates' determined negotiation of limits to night and weekend duty, privately grumbling about a declining work ethic in their profession. Some researchers echo this sentiment. Practice Sights recruiters, by contrast, attributed the focus on perks and work schedules to be a combination of naïveté and of competing opportunities in the larger job market. Anyone starting a career brings to it the hopes of Gavin Muir: good location, comfortable hours, challenging work, nice life. Those who succeed professionally usually do so because, at some level, they love the work and commit what it takes to do it well. His four-day workweek notwithstanding, Muir ended up being interviewed for this chapter at 11:00 P.M., after medical emergencies had forced him to cancel several earlier appointments. He still loves his job.

As for the larger job market, its influence was palpable during Practice Sights. Recruiters saw in many candidates a reflection of the expectations of their generational peers during a period of record-breaking prosperity in the United States. During the mid-1990s, many of the so-called best and brightest of college-educated young people flocked to quick wealth on Wall Street or in a dot com startup. The number of economics and business majors at the undergraduate level soared, while medical schools saw a precipitous drop in applicants, from a high of 46,965 in 1996 to 34,859 in 2001, according to the Association of American Medical Colleges. In this context, the emphasis on perks as opposed to the "working where I can make a difference" ethos of a previous era is less surprising—and also less predictive of future trends. It's worth noting that since Practice Sights, the dot com bubble has burst, Wall Street is laying off, and recent college graduates are beating the bushes for jobs. This is the sobering reality of today's medical school students: a context that could make job security in a medically underserved area sound very nice indeed.

That said, Practice Sights leaders identified workforce changes that are more likely to be long-term. The single-breadwinner family is becoming a rarity. Time and again, grantees found that success in recruiting and retaining providers required attention to a spouse's career or avocational interests. Married physicians are not necessarily a doctor-and-doctor package, as with David and Kari

Adams. In Littleton, New Hampshire, Jessica Thibodeau, a nurse practitioner recruited from Boston, had to be sold on the area's opportunities for her husband, Scott Brumenschenkel, a self-employed furniture maker and designer of custom cabinetry. Her job would provide the family's steady income, but for the relocation to work in the long run he needed a market for his high-end skills. Although the immediate area is poor, Thibodeau reports that Brumenschenkel was able to find customers among those with seasonal vacation homes in New Hampshire, and by way of local galleries. The couple's final concern was whether Littleton would be a good match for their school-aged daughter. The quality of the local school system was a significant draw, illustrating yet again the importance of the larger community infrastructure to health care improvements.

Another insight from Practice Sights is the need for more up-to-date and integrated national databases to guide recruiting strategies for underserved areas. The enthusiastic response of state health departments to Practice Sights stemmed in part from frustration with the disjointed status quo in health care workforce initiatives. The research field reflects this history. Much of the published data fall into isolated niches of inquiry and significantly lag behind the conditions driving decision making on the front line of recruitment and retention. The most comprehensive data sets—compiled by the federal Office of Rural Health and the Council on Graduate Medical Education—date to 1997. Any wisdom that researchers can offer a front-line recruiter is accordingly handicapped by lack of timeliness. During Practice Sights, the NPO developed computer software to assist states or small agencies in accomplishing recruiting tasks. The National Health Service Corps subsequently provided funding to make the software available to all fifty states. Similar coordination in updating and integrating disparate data sets would be helpful to those on the front line.

A final observation from the platform of Practice Sights is that there's no such thing as recruiting for permanence. Television dramas depict the silver-haired rural practitioner, beloved by his community, delivering the babies of babies he helped into the world at the start of his career. This romantic scenario is not borne out statistically. The average stay for a rural practitioner is six years. Some leave because of the specific hardships that Practice Sights sought to alleviate: long hours, isolation, and inadequate income. But others leave for the reasons that lead other professionals to jump from company to company or to move about the country: a better opportunity, family needs, or perhaps just to try something different. This mobility—part of a general workforce trend that took hold in the later years of the twentieth century—can work both ways. Rural areas occasionally benefit from providers' disenchantment with urban practice. During the 1990s, for example, California physicians left the state by the thousands rather than accept changes in practice conditions and reimbursement imposed by managed care plans. How to capitalize on the many intersecting trends and crosscurrents illustrated by Practice Sights remains a challenge for those seeking to improve access to health care in underserved communities.

Notes

1. Health Research and Services Administration, U.S. Department of Health and Human Services, "Health Professional Shortage Areas by Metropolitan/Non-Metropolitan Classification as of March 31, 2002," Table 2.
2. Rabinowitz, H., and others. "Critical Factors for Designing Programs to Increase the Supply and Retention of Rural Primary Care Physicians." *Journal of the American Medical Association*, 2001, vol. 286.
3. Marco Navarro and Peter Goodwin discuss the Foundation's PRIs in "Program-Related Investments." In *To Improve Health and Health Care. Vol. V: The Robert Wood Johnson Foundation Anthology*. San Francisco: Jossey-Bass, 2002.

4

The Foundation's End-of-Life Programs

Changing the American Way of Death

Ethan Bronner

Editors' Introduction

Since 1996, the Foundation has invested more than $148 million to improve care at the end of life. This chapter, by Ethan Bronner, an editor at the *New York Times*, takes a comprehensive look at this area of grant-making, explaining the reason the Foundation entered the field, the logic behind its strategy, and the outcomes that have emerged so far. It illustrates how a foundation can become involved in a burgeoning social movement and help give it vitality and direction.

During the 1980s and the early 1990s, Americans began to be concerned about the long period of suffering many people endured before they died. States passed laws allowing people to sign a living will, durable power of attorney, or health care proxy. Courts wrestled with issues of whether to authorize treatments that would prolong life but not restore its quality. The hospice movement became widely recognized, and hospice services were covered by Medicare. At the same time, prestigious physicians discussed, in the pages of respected medical journals, the idea that physicians should be allowed to help terminally ill patients die; Dr. Jack Kevorkian was helping people who wanted to die do so; and the Hemlock Society's book, *Final Exit*, which told readers how to commit suicide, became a best seller.

In 1988, the Foundation funded a large multi-year research study of alternate approaches to improving care at the end of life. The study found that, even with the new approaches, people still died in uncontrolled pain, hooked up to machines until just a few hours before they died; that few patients had advance directives such as a living will; and that even if they did, the directives weren't followed.[1] The results of this study led to The Robert Wood Johnson Foundation's major involvement in improving care at the end of life. (The Soros Foundation, too, has worked to improve the current culture of dying through its project on Death in America.)

At its heart, this chapter is a case study of the strategy involved in building a field by supporting thinkers, doers, and communicators who devote their professional attention to this important work. The Foundation's grantmaking in this field is generally regarded as an example of "strategic philanthropy." A small team of Foundation staff members selected three areas in which they felt the Foundation could make a difference: improving the education of practitioners; building model palliative care programs at hospitals; and raising awareness among the public. Although it is difficult to assess the success and failure of field-building efforts, the evidence presented by Bronner makes a strong case for initial success.

Perhaps what makes this area so compelling is the tension between the human and the technical. Most people who watch loved ones die after a long illness come away as advocates for improving care at the end of life and placing more emphasis on pain management. Yet this is a world with continuously emerging medical technology that can solve an increasing number of physical problems. The decision of when to switch from an all-out effort to cure a person to an effort to relieve suffering so that death can occur with comfort and dignity remains a wrenching one.

---

1. Lynn, J. "Unexpected Returns: Insights from Support." In *To Improve Health and Health Care 1997: The Robert Wood Johnson Foundation Anthology.* San Francisco: Jossey-Bass, 1997.

—ɯ— **D**iane Meier, a geriatrician at the Mount Sinai School of Medicine in New York City, was no stranger to suffering when, in 1994, she came upon something that shocked her: a seventy-three-year-old terminal cancer patient who had been strapped to his bed and force-fed for a month. Before his lung tumor metastasized to the brain and grew so large that it prevented him from speaking, the patient had repeatedly requested that no extraordinary measures be used to keep him alive. Two years earlier, he had watched his wife die of lung cancer, and under no circumstances did he wish to repeat her experience with diagnostic tests and life-prolonging treatment. He wanted to return home and die in peace.

Some months earlier, the patient had been permitted to go home, but after three grand mal seizures he was brought to the emergency room and put under the care of a new group of physicians, who pursued aggressive intervention. After he repeatedly grabbed at his feeding tube and removed it, his wrists were restrained and the tube was placed beyond his reach. That was when Diane Meier saw him. When she asked the resident on duty why the patient was being treated this way, the answer was, "Otherwise he will die." Shortly thereafter, on the twenty-ninth day of such treatment, the man's lungs and heart stopped, and he did die.

To Meier, everything about the way the man's life ended was not only tragic for him personally but also indicative of the failure of American medicine to view death in its proper context. As she and two fellow physicians at Mount Sinai, R. Sean Morrison and Christine Cassel, wrote in an article on the case in the *New England Journal of Medicine* in 1996, "The experience with this patient is a disturbing illustration of the care received by many terminally ill patients in U.S. hospitals. . . . Once an informed decision has been made to forgo life-prolonging therapy, the goal of care should be palliation. . . . It is time to ask ourselves what more can be done to relieve the suffering of patients who are dying. We need to identify the barriers to good palliative care, and address them rapidly so that this patient's experience becomes rare."[1]

In palliative care, control of pain, of other symptoms, and of psychological, social, and spiritual problems is paramount. The goal of palliative care is considered to be the best quality of life for patients and their families. This definition more closely fits the better-known and somewhat narrower concept of hospice care. The umbrella of palliative care includes hospice, which provides care for people recognized to be terminally ill and where comfort and quality of life are the only goals. But palliative care also can pursue comfort and treatment simultaneously, as in the case of patients undergoing curative treatment. (To qualify for Medicare reimbursement, hospice care requires a prognosis of death within six months; palliative care operates under no specific time frame.)

To some people, the idea of death, peaceful or otherwise, as a goal of medicine seems counterintuitive and unsettling. Medical success over the past century has been defined precisely by the myriad ways that death has been staved off. Indeed, as medical ethicist Daniel Callahan has pointed out, each technological advance that prolongs life quickly becomes routine and mandatory.[2] Yet Meier said that as she began to focus on the problem, she realized that prolonging life brings with it a new set of profound dilemmas.

"All life ends in death," Meier said one morning as she sat in her modest, packed office on the tenth floor of the Hertzberg Palliative Care Institute at Mount Sinai Hospital. "There has been an unexamined belief that with enough research, all causes of death will be defeated and we will live forever. Is this desirable? Is it good? We should also be focusing on aging gracefully. There has developed a kind of false choice: care based on maximum prolongation of life versus care based on comfort."

Meier is the director of both the Hertzberg Institute and the Center to Advance Palliative Care, which is also at Mount Sinai and funded by The Robert Wood Johnson Foundation. Meier makes another point about end-of-life care: "All surveys show that no one wants to die tethered to machinery. People want their pain controlled, they want to strengthen their relationships with family and loved ones, they want to reduce the burden on their families, and they want to complete tasks. We may steal these opportunities with technology."

—w— The Foundation's Approach to End-of-Life Programs

The Foundation's interest in this area began in 1989 when it funded a five-year study of death in hospitals. Called SUPPORT, for Study to Understand Prognoses and Preferences for Outcomes and Risks of Treatments, the $28 million study looked at nearly ten thousand critically ill patients in five major medical centers in the United States. The resulting report, published in 1995 and given wide publicity in the media, made it clear that most Americans die in hospitals, often alone and in pain, after days or weeks of futile treatment, with little advance planning, and at high cost to the institution and the family. Some patients had specified through a living will that they did not want such intervention, and many died attached to a machine in an intensive care unit. *Newsweek* summed up the findings of SUPPORT this way: "The larger problem, most analysts agree, is that American medicine lacks any concept of death as a part of life."

Commenting on SUPPORT in 1997, one of the co-investigators, Dr. Joanne Lynn, wrote, "Surely we can do better. Pain could be much more of a focus. Decisions could be made in advance, and care plans shaped much more creatively. Clearly, long-standing habits exist for a myriad of poorly understood reasons and do not yield readily to change. It may well be that change requires a much more fundamental restructuring of service supply, incentives, and rewards."[3]

Motivated by the distressing findings of SUPPORT, the Foundation, too, concluded that a major, wide-ranging effort was needed to bring attention to the importance of improving the quality of care toward the end of people's lives. It adopted a three-pronged strategy:

- *Professional education:* changing the curriculum in medical and nursing schools, modifying courses and textbooks to include end-of-life care, adding palliative care to licensure and certification examinations, training medical and nursing school faculty and practitioners, and supporting articles for professional journals such as the *Journal of the American Medical Association* and the *American Journal of Nursing*

- *Institutional change:* building palliative care capacity in the nation's hospitals, where more than half of Americans die; working with hospital accreditation agencies to develop pain management standards; and stimulating innovative programs that provide palliative care

- *Public engagement:* creating a new vision of end-of-life care through the media (both information and entertainment), and getting individuals and communities to take action to improve care for dying people and their families

The strategy has a logical flow. "We're trying to change the attitude of the medical and nursing community," says Rosemary Gibson, a senior program officer at the Foundation who chairs its end-of-life team. "Without their support, little will happen. But it's not enough. We've got to institutionalize palliative care by making it a normal part of medical and nursing care of seriously ill patients and by creating centers of excellence. And we've got to go farther; we've got to change the culture of American society. What we're really trying to do is make this mainstream—to make it part of the nation's genetic code."

It seems paradoxical that as technology prolongs life, a movement should take root that focuses on accepting death and improving the care given to dying people. Researchers say that interest in palliative care has arisen now because of several intersecting factors. The first is demographic. People in the baby boom generation—the postwar population bulge—have come face-to-face in recent years with the lackluster care given their parents as they age and die. The second reason for the new attention is the focus on physician-assisted suicide that has been created by Dr. Jack Kevorkian in the late 1980s and the 1990s, by an Oregon law permitting it, and by a U.S. Supreme Court decision adjudicating it. Third was the unequivocal nature of SUPPORT's findings, confirming everyone's worst fears about the kind of care Americans receive. Finally, advocates say, a number of doctors and nurses in their forties and fifties who were becoming disillusioned with their profession because of managed care's growing emphasis on the bottom line found in palliative care a source of renewed inspiration. Together, these factors have created the seeds of change. But shifting something as fundamental as how Americans die will not be simple or quick. According to Vicki Weisfeld, a Robert Wood Johnson Foundation senior communications officer and member of the Foundation's end-of-life team:

> Our biggest enemy is the status quo. Nobody wants to torture dying people, yet everyone has had these experiences. They come away thinking, 'I don't want anyone else to go through what my mother went through,' or 'If only everyone could have as peaceful a passing as Aunt Tilly.' But everyone interprets the experience as a totally idiosyncratic confluence of disease, personality, doctor, and so on. They don't see it as reflecting systemic issues. But it is. We are trying to be catalysts, to get people to start paying attention, to create the conditions so that in ten to fif-

teen years end-of-life care will be seen not as a separate entity but as a logical extension of chronic care.

—⁓— Changing the Attitudes of Health Professionals

Changing a system requires, as much as anything, changing the views and practices of its leaders and practitioners—in this case, the members of the medical and nursing professions. The Robert Wood Johnson Foundation has focused part of its funding of end-of-life care on modifying how doctors and nurses are trained. This is vital because, as George Annas, a Boston University law professor and medical ethicist, has argued, "Physicians simply have never taken the rights of hospitalized patients seriously. The central reason is that in the modern teaching hospital, patient care is often a distant third goal after teaching and research. In the high-tech, high-pressure environment, there is little room for thoughtfulness, for the intrusion of human values, or for conversation with the patient or family."[4]

In 1998, the Foundation gave $832,000 to Stanford University and $998,000 to Massachusetts General Hospital to provide in-depth training to medical school faculty so they are equipped to teach end-of-life care to their students and other faculty members. Stanford trains medical faculty members from across the country in a month-long program, and the people it trains then act as resources for faculty members and others in their home institution. The grant to Massachusetts General Hospital helped jump start the Center for Palliative Care at the Harvard Medical School, which trains physicians and nurse educators to become expert—and to train others—in the clinical practice and teaching of comprehensive, interdisciplinary palliative care.

With funding from The Robert Wood Johnson Foundation, Tom Bowles, president of the National Board of Medical Examiners, took on the task of increasing the quantity and quality of end-of-life questions on the U.S. Medical Licensing Examination. David Weissman, professor of internal medicine at the Medical College of Wisconsin, has been working to overcome the core barriers to training regarding end-of-life care in the residency setting. Among the projects carried out under his Robert Wood Johnson Foundation grant was a one-year pilot program for thirty residency programs in the Midwest; it has subsequently attracted nearly two hundred residency programs. The Foundation has also funded a program to train practicing physicians, called Education for Physicians on End-of-Life Care. The training sessions have consistently been oversubscribed, and the training materials are in great demand.

The Foundation also gave out grants to assess how medical textbooks treat end-of-life care. Stephen McPhee, a physician at the University of California, San Francisco, School of Medicine and director of the medical textbook project, said that leading medical textbooks were markedly deficient in end-of-life issues. Chapters on fatal diseases focus on prognosis and are rarely concerned with treating symptoms, decision making about terminal care, and the impact of death on a patient's family.

McPhee and his colleagues carried out a study of medical textbooks. They set up categories of topics that should be covered, among them epidemiology, natural history, pain management, psychological issues such as depression and fear, and social and demographic issues as well as cultural and spiritual ones. The results were published in the *Journal of the American Medical Association*.[5] The investigators reported that, overall, helpful information was found in about 24 percent of those categories. In more than 56 percent of them, discussion of relevant end-of-life topics was entirely absent.

More than a year later, McPhee and his colleagues reported on follow-up they carried out with editors and publishers.[6] They found that of the fifty leading medical textbooks, more than one-third were planning to expand or had already expanded end-of-life care content in their next edition. They also received six personal letters from editors and publishers supportive of the project, including a poignant one from a textbook editor who was himself dying of cancer at the time he wrote. Meanwhile, as McPhee pointed out in his follow-up, much work remains to be done. Most best-selling textbooks, including oncology (cancer) and hematology (blood diseases) texts, have not responded to the suggestions of their specialty board and others to improve clinical education in end-of-life care.

Of course, training doctors only goes so far. Nurses actually provide most of the care to the dying, and in nursing homes, where a growing proportion of people die, nurses provide almost all of the professional services. So the Foundation is funding a high-quality palliative care training program for nurses, attempting to increase the attention given to palliative care in the nursing school curriculum, analyzing and trying to improve how nursing textbooks treat end-of-life issues,[7] and working to have end-of-life care made a part of the nurse licensing exams.

—⨯⨯— Bringing Palliative Care into the Medical Mainstream

To institutionalize palliative care and make it a normal part of the care of gravely ill patients, the Foundation has worked to create a more hospitable environment for it in the nation's health care facilities. It has given out a range of grants to bring about institutional change. Two of the more compelling are an award to Mount Sinai Medical Center in New York City to establish the Center to Advance Palliative Care, which focuses on integrating palliative care into hospitals, and an award to the Practical Ethics Center of the University of Montana, Missoula, for a program called Promoting Excellence in End-of-Life Care, with the goal of encouraging innovative demonstration projects to improve care for dying patients.

Mount Sinai's Palliative Care Unit

A meeting of the palliative care unit at Mount Sinai at 8:00 A.M. on a November morning illustrates one of the approaches supported by the Foundation. Seven specialists—a social worker, a nurse practitioner, two nurses, and three doctors—gather in the office of Jane Morris, a nurse who is the unit's clinical coordinator, for the weekly meeting. They examine a list of ten very ill patients, most of whom are elderly. There is also a thirty-two-year-old male with a failed intestinal transplant and a forty-year-old male with hepatitis C. Coffee cups sit alongside clipboards; the high pitch of beepers frequently interrupts the discussion. A sense of camaraderie and shared mission pervades the room.

"Miss K. is a seventy-four-year-old with hypertension and dementia," Tim McGrath, the nurse practitioner, tells his colleagues. "She has three sons and all are on their way here because she recently attempted suicide."

"What about her pain?" asks Diane Meier, the group's leader. "Does she have pressure sores? She's a very large woman who has been in bed a very long time."

In this as in other cases, drug doses and therapies are discussed and debated. Often the question comes up: Has she made her wishes known?

After the meeting, McGrath goes to the gastrointestinal care center to check on a number of patients. He focuses on their comfort and personal and human needs rather than on the progress of their medical therapies. His first stop is Don Koll, a seventy-eight-year-old retired actor who has carcinoid syndrome, meaning that he suffers from a web of related symptoms, such as cramps and diarrhea, caused by tumors in his digestive track. A once-strapping 5'10" and 190 pounds, Koll is down to 140. Having earned a good living from advertisements of, among other things, Swift Butterball turkeys (he was the handsome, kindly looking father who told his wife that the turkey was "really juicy"), Koll today can't keep his food down. It is a cruel paradox, of which Koll is aware. McGrath asks about his walking.

"I still can only go so far and then I have to sit and pant," comes the matter-of-fact reply. They also discuss where Koll should go when leaving the hospital.

After McGrath moves on to other patients, Koll speaks of the value of his visit: "I'm prone to depression, so it helps me when they come around to talk like this," he said. "The rest of the staff here on the ward are really too busy to do it, so it is good to have these palliative care folks come. I'll be leaving here in a few days, and they are helping me make those arrangements."

Some minutes later, McGrath is on the telephone at the nurses' station talking with a member of a Hispanic family in the Bronx that wants to bring back their mother, who has liver cancer.

"What do they hope to accomplish by bringing her into the hospital?" McGrath asks, speaking to a family member whose English is fluent. "The IV fluid is not going to change things. Our goal is to keep her at home and comfortable as long as possible."

The children decide to bring their mother in anyway, in the faint hope that her condition will improve in the hospital.

Promoting Excellence in End-of-Life Care

In 1997, the $12-million Promoting Excellence in End-of-Life Care program, based at the University of Montana, Missoula, issued a call for creative strategies for delivering palliative care in difficult clinical contexts. Some 678 letters of intent arrived from fifty states and two territories. After an intense review process, twenty-two projects were chosen, each funded for up to $450,000 over three years. The three broad priority areas were (1) special populations, including children, Native Americans, the seriously mentally ill, and urban African Americans; (2) specific diseases and conditions, including Alzheimer's and advanced HIV; and (3) challenging clinical settings, such as nursing homes, cancer centers, rural communities, and maximum-security prisons. The aim of the projects is to build models that can be sustained and adopted more widely. Jeanne Twohig, the deputy director of Promoting Excellence, says that in many of those projects that aim is being realized.

Among the special populations receiving support are Alaskan Natives served by the Bristol Bay Area Health Corporation. The project has been dubbed Ikayurtem Unatai, which in Yup'ik means Helping Hands; it aims at providing end-of-life care to thirty-two villages throughout a Bristol Bay area of forty-seven thousand square-miles. Village leaders say they have been unhappy that terminally ill elders are often flown to a hospital hundreds of miles away in Dillingham or Anchorage, where they spend the last days of their lives and die far from village and family.

"They knew that when an elder was sick they would probably never see the person again, and that caused a lot of trauma," said Christine DeCourtney, who helped establish and run the program for three years and who remains a consultant in Dillingham. "The program has proved very popular. The families are now more involved in care. It used to be that 33 percent were dying in the villages. Now it is 77 percent." Twohig added:

> When someone is about to die, they have what amounts to a town meeting to provide volunteers so the person can die at home. They have produced a brochure in Yup'ik for volunteers, which talks about issues specific to their culture such as helping families dry their berries and hang their fish. Now that patients are staying

at home, there is a huge cost saving, because they are not airlifting them, and there is real improvement in grief and bereavement. And the project is being picked up by the Alaskan Native Tribal Health Consortium in Anchorage to spread it across the twelve different native regions.

In essence, DeCourtney explained, the program returns death to the place it had for centuries in Yup'ik culture, but with the addition of Western medicine to reduce pain and of case managers and social workers to reduce anxiety.

Although about 85 percent of whites generally say they wish to die at home, the numbers are different for Latinos and African Americans. About a third of both Latinos and blacks say they do not want to die at home, according to Dr. Jerome Kurent, an associate professor of medicine at the Medical University of South Carolina, another grant recipient. Among the reasons given for preferring to die in a hospital, he said, were that better care and equipment were available there and that some members of the community are not comfortable continuing to live in a house where someone has died.

Much about the difference in group attitude toward pain and dying is unexplored, but there is a body of research that speaks of broad differences among groups. "We've come very far in defining what a good death means for most white, middle-class Americans," says Dr. Leslie Blackhall of the University of Virginia's Center for Biomedical Ethics. "But we have to be careful that we don't project those ideas on people from different cultural backgrounds who may want more lifesaving technology than we would want, who may not want to make all the decisions."[8]

There is also research indicating that those in racial and ethnic minorities in the United States lack access to treatment for pain, and that this may contribute to their desire to go to the hospital when very ill. Contributing factors include physicians' reluctance to prescribe (and patients' reluctance to use) powerful medication, fear of addiction, and the high cost of drugs. In addition, preliminary evidence indicates that pharmacies in neighborhoods where most residents are not white are less likely to carry opioids than pharmacies in predominantly white neighborhoods.[9]

To promote greater education in end-of-life issues in South Carolina, Kurent and his team engaged ministers in the community, who went through some twenty hours of workshops on care options and issues of spirituality, taboo, and myth. Among the issues discussed was pain management. Kurent said some elderly members of the community considered pain upon dying to be God's wish, or even punishment, and that sensitive discussion of pain among the dying was, therefore, essential.

In Birmingham, Alabama, the Balm of Gilead, another grant recipient, seeks to integrate existing acute care and end-of-life care throughout Jefferson County and to identify patients who need help earlier. It focuses on medically underserved people with terminal illnesses who have no place to live or need support services at home.

Balm of Gilead provides palliative care at a dedicated ten-bed unit on the fourth floor of Cooper Green Hospital. Each room is furnished and decorated in homelike fashion by a local church or community group. Throughout the hospital, Balm of Gilead promotes the idea of addressing pain as a fifth vital sign and has introduced advance directives into the hospital and its clinics so that patients' wishes are known prior to admission. Since such directives were not widely used by the patients served by the hospital, the staff developed an interview script for use when speaking with patients and families. This has resulted in a much higher rate of acceptance of those documents, says Balm of Gilead's director, F. Amos Bailey. According to The Robert Wood Johnson Foundation's Rosemary Gibson, the project has stimulated five other hospitals in Birmingham, among them the University of Alabama at Birmingham, to establish palliative care programs.

—⚭— Changing Public Attitudes

Public education is central to changing Americans' expectations about the kind of care seriously ill patients should receive, and the Foundation has invested in a variety of initiatives aimed at increasing knowledge and shifting popular attitudes.

Last Acts® is a campaign of more than nine hundred partner organizations working to change the public's attitude toward end-of-life care. Former first lady Rosalynn Carter serves as its honorary chairwoman. Last Acts holds national and regional conferences about end-of-life care, works with policy makers and the media, publishes a quarterly newsletter, and has established a Website (www.lastacts.org). Among Last Acts' publications are definitions of palliative care (endorsed by more than 150 groups), a series of policy briefs, and a sheet with suggestions of what to do if you or someone you love is very ill. It offers guidelines for questions to ask of the doctor ("If I reach a point where I am too sick to speak for myself, how will you make decisions about my care?"), the family ("Will you respect my wants and needs, even if they're different from what they used to be, or if you think they are strange or silly?"), and the clergy ("If I have negative feelings like frustration, sadness, despair, anger at God or life, will you listen empathetically?").

Last Acts includes a Writers Project, based in Los Angeles. Run by Bill Duke, a former newspaperman and longtime public relations professional, the project has, since 1998, made end-of-life experts and plot lines available to script writers and producers of television dramas. Several of its story ideas have appeared within episodes of the highly popular NBC series "ER" and others in programs such as "Gideon's Crossing," "NYPD Blue," and "City of Angels." In two late-2000 episodes of "ER," the death of Dr. Green's father explored the emotional as well as the medical needs of the dying.

Duke also worked with HBO on the Mike Nichols version (filmed in Great Britain) of the Pulitzer Prize–winning Broadway play "Wit," starring Emma Thompson, about a sharp-tongued professor dying of ovarian cancer. Last Acts made a technical expert available on the set to be sure the show accurately depicted hospital care around 1990.

"Some people ask how we evaluate our effectiveness," Duke said, "and that is a fair question. We are not dealing here with something as straightforward as product placement. We are dealing with ideas. But I can tell you this: until this year, I hadn't ever heard phrases such as 'palliative care' used on television." Duke added, "By watching these shows, people may have received their first exposure to how terminal illness is treated today and what they can do to make their final days more comfortable—more emotionally satisfying."

The Foundation's single biggest investment in public education, some $2.75 million, was in cosponsoring a widely viewed and critically acclaimed, four-part, six-hour PBS documentary with Bill Moyers on dying in America, called "On Our Own Terms." Julie Salomon, the television critic of the *New York Times*, called it "an extraordinary guide" and "panoramic and often profoundly moving."

Shown across the country in September 2000 and viewed by twenty million people, the series opened with Moyers speaking directly to the viewers:

> Like you, I don't want to think about death, especially my own. But I've realized that death is pushing through the door we try to keep so firmly shut. Parents age before our eyes. AIDS and cancer take friends and loved ones. And baby boomers, that most powerful generation in our culture, face their own mortality even as they care for their aging parents. So, like it or not, we can't push death back through the door. That's one reason we did this series. The other is that there is a movement afoot driven by our hope for a better death.

The series took the viewers on what it called "intimate journeys of the dying." The first episode, called "Living with Dying," focused on Bill Bartholome, a Kansas City pediatrician in his fifties with three daughters, who has terminal cancer of the esophagus. He decides to stay away from chemotherapy and other aggressive anti-cancer treatments and keeps a journal on the months and years that end in his death. Bartholome tells Moyers that living in the light of dying offers an entirely new perspective on life, one through which the song of the meadowlark or the arrival of spring is infused with significance. It is a lesson, he says, that he wished he had understood and appreciated before it was forced on him by his diagnosis. Viewers watch as he, his daughters, and his fiancée prepare for his death at home, where he is surrounded by their love. Other stories, called "A Different Kind of Care," "A Death of One's Own," and "A Time to Change," explore elements of the same point: the choices people have that can lead to a more peaceful death.

The broadcast was linked to a Website that encouraged further exploration. During the program, the screen highlighted what could be found there, including information on both practical and intangible matters, such as financial planning for terminally ill patients, various treatment alternatives, and "taking a spiritual inventory."

In conjunction with the series, the Foundation supported community outreach, hoping to spur about one hundred communities to take action locally. In fact, more than three hundred had some form of town meeting or other activity.

To bring about policy and regulatory change at the state and local levels, the Foundation funded a national program called Community-State Partnerships to Improve End-of-Life Care. Administered through the Midwest Bioethics

Center in Kansas City, Missouri, the program awarded grants to promote policy change and support for high-quality, comprehensive palliative care in some twenty-one states, from Hawaii to Maine. The projects typically involve forming a broad-based coalition that determines priority issues, collects data, develops an action plan, promotes community discussion, suggests ways to improve palliative care, and fosters dialogue within a religious community. In Kentucky, for example, Kentuckians for Compassionate Care, a partnership of more than fifty agencies, is identifying strategies to increase awareness among physicians, nurses, and the public about end-of-life care. Among its many activities, it has established a peer resource network and a toll-free help line for consultation and support to clinicians having difficulty managing pain and other symptoms in their terminally ill patients.

—⟋⟍— Conclusions

Palliative care comprises a number of elements—managing symptoms, communication between families and professional caregivers, spiritual and emotional support—but many consider pain management to be the first priority. A 1997 report by the Institute of Medicine emphasized that the number one fear that dying people had was the possibility of being in excruciating pain.[10] Although experts say that pain can be controlled effectively in 90–95 percent of patients, each year a large number of Americans suffer pain unnecessarily as they die.

Palliative care proponents seek not only redefinition of appropriate end-of-life care but also shifted consciousness about the role of pain in medicine more broadly. This means measuring patient discomfort as a legitimate and standard practice as well as teaching health care providers the least intrusive and least painful ways to carry out various standard procedures.

A shift in the medical profession's attitude toward pain has, in fact, begun. In 1999, with funding from The Robert Wood Johnson Foundation, the Joint Commission on Accreditation of Healthcare Organizations, which accredits the majority of the country's medical facilities, developed new mandatory standards for assessing and treating pain. By January 2001, surveyors began scoring pain management programs and applying the results in the accreditation process. In 1999, the Oregon

Board of Medical Examiners disciplined a pulmonary specialist for undertreating severe pain (for example, by refusing to prescribe morphine to an eighty-two-year-old with congestive heart failure). The board ruled that the physician had shown unprofessional conduct and gross and repeated negligence in undertreating six seriously ill or dying patients. From the point of view of palliative care advocates, this shift is a good beginning. But the goal is larger: to make pain a fifth vital sign along with temperature, pulse, respiration, and blood pressure; and to get medical schools and residency programs to focus on the pain experienced by patients.

It is too early to say if the changes more generally sought by those hoping to improve end-of-life care will come about before the Foundation ends its substantial investment. But it is not too early to say that much has already been achieved in a short time:

- Surveys in 2001 from the American Hospital Association and the Center to Advance Palliative Care indicated that over 300 hospitals had palliative care programs, and more than 200 were planning to establish one.[11] This represents a relatively small percentage of the six thousand hospitals in the United States, but the growth has all occurred in recent years.

- The Last Acts campaign developed "precepts" for what good palliative care includes, such as respecting patients' choices and providing comprehensive (including spiritual and emotional) care to patients and their families. The precepts have been endorsed by 162 organizations, as of May 2002.

- The National Cancer Policy Board of the Institute of Medicine recently stated that palliative care should be an integral part of good quality cancer care.

There is little doubt that palliative care and new approaches to understanding death have become legitimized quickly. As Judith Miller, a *New York Times* reporter, put it in a 1997 article on work by the Soros Foundation and The Robert Wood Johnson Foundation in this area, "Foundation giving has often helped create academic and public interest in a topic. . . . But the sharp increase in research on death demonstrates the growing power of philanthropy almost to create an academic field."[12]

Notes

1. Morrison, R. S., Meier, D. E., and Cassel, C. K. "When Too Much Is Too Little." *New England Journal of Medicine,* 1996, vol. 335, p. 1755.

2. Callahan, D. *The Troubled Dream of Life: Living with Mortality.* New York: Simon & Schuster, 1993.

3. Lynn, J. "Unexpected Returns: Insights from SUPPORT." In *To Improve Health and Health Care 1997: The Robert Wood Johnson Foundation Anthology.* San Francisco: Jossey-Bass, 1997.

4. "Hastings Center Report Supplement," Nov.–Dec. 1995, p. S12.

5. Rabow, M. W., Hardie, G. E., Fair, J. M., and McPhee, S. J. "End-of-Life Care Content in 50 Textbooks from Multiple Specialties." *Journal of the American Medical Association,* 2000, *283*(6), 771–778.

6. Rabow, M. W., and McPhee, S. J. "Patients' Needs at the End of Life." *Journal of Clinical Oncology,* 2001, *19*(15), 3585.

7. See, for example, Ferrell, B. R. "Analysis of Symptom Assessment and Management Content in Nursing Textbooks." *Journal of Palliative Medicine,* 1999, *2,* 161–172.

8. Quoted in Carey, B. "Last Days Needn't Be Spent in Agony." *Los Angeles Times,* Aug. 20, 2001.

9. Gibson, R. "For Richer or for Poorer: Palliative Care for the Poor and Disenfranchised and the Role of Philanthropic Organizations." Paper prepared for the Palliative Care Conference of the Royal Society of Medicine, London, Dec. 11–12, 2000, rev. Apr. 5, 2001.

10. Institute of Medicine, Committee on Care at the End of Life, *Approaching Death*, Field, M. J., and Cassel, C.K. (eds.). Washington, DC: National Academy Press, 1997.

11. Pan, C. X., and others. "How Prevalent Are Hospital-Based Palliative Care Programs? Status Report and Future Directions." *Journal of Palliative Medicine,* 2001, *4*(3), 307–308.

12. Miller, J. "When Foundations Chime In, the Issue of Dying Comes to Life." *New York Times,* Nov. 22, 1997.

Improving Health

5

The Center for Tobacco-Free Kids and the Tobacco-Settlement Negotiations

Digby Diehl

Editors' Introduction

The Center for Tobacco-Free Kids was created in 1995 to develop and promote a national strategy to reduce smoking by young people and to be a focal point for communicating with the media. Soon after it was established, an unprecedented set of circumstances created a unique opportunity for the Center to become involved in the comprehensive legal settlement that was being negotiated between the tobacco industry and state governments. While the Center carried out—and continues to carry out—a broad range of policy, communications, advocacy, and technical support activities, its involvement in the tobacco negotiations thrust it into a role far different than the one it played previously or subsequently.

In this chapter, Digby Diehl, a free-lance writer and frequent contributor to *The Robert Wood Johnson Foundation Anthology* series, tells the story of this exceptional 15-month period in the Center's history. The Center's involvement in the tobacco settlement was controversial. Indeed, the anti-tobacco community was fragmented, and its members disagreed about the role the Center should play in the negotiations, the wisdom of sitting down with the tobacco companies, and the terms of the settlement itself.

As it turned out, Congress did not approve the settlement, the states that had been suing the tobacco companies agreed to a watered-down version, and the Center moved on to support the efforts of state and local advocates to improve the resources at their disposal, to work with them to bring professional communications skills to the effort, and to develop plans to reach out to communities not previously involved in tobacco work.

Was the Center's role effective in a process that did not succeed when the political forces failed to align in the end? Was the Center a central part of a flawed process? Was its role appropriate, or did it overreach in becoming a key part of the negotiations? Definitive answers to these questions are not possible. But the story describing the efforts of the Center and the thinking of its leaders can shed light on the questions. Diehl provides an outsider's review in this chapter; it complements an insider's review by Michael Pertschuk in a recent book (partially funded by The Robert Wood Johnson Foundation) titled *Smoke in Their Eyes.*[1]

Although the Foundation's $70 million investment in the Center for Tobacco-Free Kids is substantial, the grants to the Center represent just 17 percent of the approximately $408 million that the Foundation has committed to efforts to reduce tobacco use. The overall Foundation strategy, which has focused largely on getting children to stop (or not start) smoking, has been a comprehensive one: supporting research to improve understanding of why young people smoke and what interventions would reduce their use of tobacco; training professionals interested in advocating against tobacco use; financing public policy analysis to assess the pros and cons of public interventions to reduce tobacco use among young people; working with states on ways to reduce smoking among young people; and funding demonstrations of new approaches to tobacco cessation.[2]

1. Pertschuk, M. *Smoke in Their Eyes: Lessons in Movement Leadership From the Tobacco Wars.* Nashville: Vanderbuilt University, 2001.

2. Other chapters of *The Robert Wood Johnson Foundation Anthology* examining the Foundation's work to curb tobacco use are Hughes, R. G. "Adopting the Substance Abuse Goal: A Story of Philanthropic Decision Making" (1998–99); Kaufman, N. J., and Feiden, K. L. "Linking Biomedical and Behavioral Research for Tobacco Use Prevention: Sundance and Beyond" (2000); and Chapter Six in this volume, by C. Tracy Orleans and Joseph Alper.

**Attract a smoker at the earliest opportunity and
let brand loyalty turn that smoker into a valuable
asset.**

Internal R. J. Reynolds marketing memo,
"Strategies and Segments,"
from R. C. Nordine to E. J. Fackelman
April 13, 1984[1]

—W— Since World War I, when truckloads of free cigarettes were distributed to American soldiers by the U.S. government, millions of Americans have been addicted to tobacco products. Despite tobacco's tragic role as a leading health hazard, for many years public health organizations were reluctant to address it. The seemingly intractable core of the problem was that for adults, tobacco use is not against the law. More significant—although rarely mentioned openly—most health advocates were afraid of the powerful corporations that manufactured and marketed cigarettes, as well as the formidable political forces in Congress and elsewhere that were supported by tobacco industry lobbies.

—W— The Genesis of the Center for Tobacco-Free Kids

Upon arriving at The Robert Wood Johnson Foundation as president in 1990, Steven Schroeder encouraged the board and the staff to confront the tremendous public health damage of tobacco. Not long ago he said:

> When I interviewed with the Foundation board, I told them I thought the Foundation should get more involved with substance abuse—that they were missing an opportunity. When I told the staff members that, and asked them to think about it, they didn't want to do tobacco. Ultimately, the staff came around, and our board members felt the same way, but they were worried about the power of the legal

industries, the alcohol and the tobacco industries, to resist what we might do and to make things ugly for us—to sully the good name of The Robert Wood Johnson Foundation.

When we proposed to go at this issue, we had a very spirited debate on the board. We actually had an eight-to-eight tie, with some board members thumping the table saying, "We shouldn't do this; we're a health care foundation." Fortunately, the mission of the Foundation is health care *and* health. By being able to bring the question back to the mission and the data, we were able to break the tie.

What also helped to break the stalemate was some creative thinking by one of the trustees. Because reluctant board members were deeply troubled by the legality of tobacco use, the trustee suggested placing the focus on underage smokers—for whom tobacco use was and is against the law. With the legal issue thus resolved, the board endorsed that thrust. In 1991, the Foundation awarded a grant to Stop Teenage Addictions to Tobacco. Two years later, it began funding the SmokeLess States® National Tobacco Policy Initiative. Now almost a decade old, SmokeLess States continues to fund development and implementation of statewide strategies to reduce tobacco usage through education, treatment, and public policy. Among other techniques, the program seeks to increase the excise tax on cigarettes and the number of places having a smoke-free environmental policy.

A different approach to grappling with smoking on the national level came later, taking shape in Paris at the ninth World Conference on Tobacco and Health in October of 1994. Held every three years, this conference is part postgraduate seminar on sources and methods to combat smoking addiction and part old-time-religion tent revival intended to rally and energize the faithful. Foundation vice president Nancy Kaufman, who had been hired in 1991 for her background in public health and substance abuse, was part of The Robert Wood Johnson Foundation delegation to the conference. "People involved in tobacco control come to these conferences from all over the world," she says. "Some are academics, some work for governments, and some are true on-the-ground advocates who are not professionally trained in health at all. At that meeting in Paris, I was bowled over. I saw all this incredible tobacco control activity going on in other countries. We looked like we were in the Stone Age by comparison."

At that conference, Kaufman brought together a dedicated group of tobacco control advocates to try to figure out what the antismoking movement in the United States could do to catch up with its more assertive and innovative foreign counterparts. Included in the group of Americans in Paris were Matt Myers, a Washington anti-tobacco attorney; John Bloom, a lawyer and consultant for the National Cancer Society; John Slade, a physician and professor at the University of Medicine and Dentistry of New Jersey; Greg Connolly, director of the tobacco control program for the state of Massachusetts; and Michael Beachler, then a senior program officer at The Robert Wood Johnson Foundation. The group gathered between sessions of the conference, and the idea of a national center—a home base for the antismoking movement—began to form.

The germ of this idea had already been planted in a Foundation study conducted by Elaine Arkin earlier in 1994.[2] "We hired Elaine Arkin to surf for ideas that would improve communication and education efforts that would denormalize tobacco," says Beachler, who is now the director of Penn State's Rural Health Policy Center. Arkin talked with a great many of the experts in the field, synthesized their ideas, and brought them to the Foundation's attention. "She came back with a series of options, one of which was a national center that would act as a central clearinghouse—*the* place where tobacco opponents could congregate to create their message. What we ended up doing was different, but her work put the idea of a national center on the horizon."

The Tobacco Institute was the public relations arm of the tobacco industry. Armed with a multimillion dollar budget and using a combination of savvy Washington political maneuvering and sophisticated advertising and public relations campaigns, the Institute sought to manipulate public opinion on smoking and to counter claims that smoking is unhealthy and potentially deadly.[3] For more than four decades, despite the mounting scientific evidence on the adverse health effects of smoking cigarettes, it was remarkably successful.[4] The problem was that although the Tobacco Institute offered the media one-stop shopping for the pro-tobacco spin on events and information, there wasn't just one place journalists could go for a rebuttal. Anti-tobacco forces were fragmented across numerous public health and public interest organizations, and opposition to the tobacco lobby was not the sole mission of any of them—"Tobacco was just one more item on a long list of issues these organizations cared about. We were like guerrillas, firing spears and darts at panzer tanks," says Joe Marx, currently a senior communications officer for The Robert Wood Johnson Foundation who, at the time, directed media relations for the American Heart Association.

To the extent that they were organized at all, the anti-tobacco "guerrillas" worked out of the Coalition on Smoking OR Health, a loose confederation of representatives of the American Cancer Society, the American Lung Association, and the American Heart Association. "The overriding weakness of the coalition was that it was rather an exclusive club," says Beachler, "and it was limited in what it could bring to the table in terms of organizational and political muscle. What was needed was a big tent of people who could really push and mobilize on a specific issue."

Moreover, the Coalition on Smoking OR Health was strapped for resources. "The Coalition never had the resources to do the job" says Matt Myers, a former civil rights attorney who was executive director of the Coalition and is now president of the National Center for Tobacco Free Kids. The Coalition responded to legislation proposed by Big Tobacco and to the industry's media blitzes, but only rarely did it initiate activities of its own.

The idea of having a national center with not just a communications focus but also a policy-making edge took shape at those informal meetings in Paris. The challenge was how to create an organization that would seize the initiative and function as a Tobacco Institute for the good guys. The concept of being proactive was to be a giant step forward. Not only would the center serve the press, providing information, documentation, and sound bites for the anti-tobacco point of view, it would also work for measures to denormalize tobacco.

Shortly after the Paris conference, Kaufman and Beachler met with Steven Schroeder and proposed the idea of a new organization. With a green light from Schroeder, the pair began putting it together. The concept was not without risk. For The Robert Wood Johnson Foundation at that time, tobacco control was a controversial activity.

Although the Foundation's antismoking activities in the early 1990s had been modest, they had not gone unnoticed by the tobacco industry, which had already fired one warning shot across the bow, over the SmokeLess States program. To gear up for a public-health-oriented series of TV commercials concerning smoking and children, the Foundation's grantee in Colorado had held an open bidders' conference for firms interested in producing the ads. Although a tobacco tax referendum on raising the state tax on a pack of cigarettes was to go before Colorado voters in the fall of 1994, the proposed public health messages had nothing to do with cigarette taxes. Nevertheless, a tobacco industry lawyer attended the bidders' conference, and reported back to the Washington law firm of Covington & Burling, long affiliated with the tobacco industry. Covington & Burling sent an intimidating letter to The Robert Wood Johnson Foundation, alleging that the Foundation was using its money illegally, and threatening IRS involvement.

Although the Colorado public health campaign was surely an aggressive use of Foundation funds, staff members had ascertained beforehand that any use of grant monies would stay nonpolitical. Nevertheless, the letter from Covington & Burling generated considerable anxiety when it arrived, as Michael Beachler recalls:

> The letter hit the Foundation doorstep about three weeks before we were to make a presentation to the board about launching what would become Tobacco-Free Kids. We had to make the fact that we'd gotten this semithreatening letter from the tobacco industry part of the presentation. We crafted a strategy that reassured the trustees that the Foundation knew what it was doing, and that we were on the right side of the law. We also made it perfectly clear that no Robert Wood Johnson Foundation funds could be used for lobbying.

The Foundation did not, however, want to support this new organization all by itself. For political and symbolic reasons, it needed other partners at the table that believed this was an important concept. It contacted the leadership of the American Cancer Society, the American Heart Association, and the American Lung Association—organizations that were the nucleus of the Coalition on Smoking OR Health—as well as with other activists in the public health community. With their moral support and the financial the backing of the American Cancer Society and the American Heart Association, in September of 1995 The Robert Wood Johnson Foundation provided funding for a coordinating committee that would eventually become the nucleus of the National Center for

Tobacco-Free Kids. The project began on a hope and a shoestring—and on the serendipitous availability of William D. Novelli.

~∿~ The Center Takes Wing

A founder of the Washington, D.C., social marketing firm of Porter Novelli, Bill Novelli had been in the number-two position at CARE, but had just left to take a sabbatical at the Annenberg Center at the University of Pennsylvania. He was all but literally pen-in-hand, ready to sign a year's lease in Philadelphia in connection with his teaching position, but it didn't take much cajoling for him to change his plans and become the first president of the National Center for Tobacco-Free Kids. What would make someone give up the comfort of a visiting professorship? As Novelli says:

> The sabbatical was going to be a real respite—I was going to take a course, teach a course, drink some beer, and go to football games. Then Dr. Tom Houston of the American Medical Association called to tell me that the Food and Drug Administration was about to assert jurisdiction over tobacco, and that we needed to get something going. Shortly thereafter, Nancy Kaufman called and offered me the presidency of the Center for Tobacco-Free Kids. I saw this as a major opportunity to really make a difference, to tackle something that had a huge, huge payoff. That was number one. Number two, the tobacco industry is the kind of entity that really gets your juices flowing.
>
> The third thing was that when I retired from Porter Novelli, I told myself that I was going to really go for the gold. I wanted to have opportunities to work with great people and do great things. I said to myself, "This will be a hell of a lot more fun than a sabbatical. This will be a great fight."

Shortly after Labor Day in 1995, with borrowed office space and what was literally a skeleton crew, Novelli began gearing up for battle with the tobacco industry. The battle was surely coming—just the month before, the White House and the Food and Drug Administration announced their intention to assert jurisdiction over tobacco. Although the Center for Tobacco-Free Kids was still in its infancy, the organization had already registered as a blip on Big Tobacco's radar.

"They play hardball," Novelli says. "Within a month of when I started, there was a blurb about me in the *Wall Street Journal*, about Bill Novelli coming back to Washington to run Tobacco-Free Kids. About a week later, I got a call from a guy who was working at a PR agency that services Philip Morris. He said, 'Bill, they're doing a dossier on you. They're asking all kinds of questions.' "

Big Tobacco was also shaken by a series of paid advertisements that the Center took out starting in the fall of 1995. "We wanted to create as much public outrage as we could," Novelli says. "We wanted to isolate the tobacco industry from the standpoint of their role in corporate America, and not make them seem like just another corporation or industry." Says Matt Myers, who officially joined the Center as vice president at the launch in June, 1996 and became president in 1999 when Bill Novelli resigned to head the AARP:

> This was the first time that the tobacco control movement had the ability to buy advertising, and it put the world on notice that Tobacco-Free Kids existed. The ads were remarkably successful.

In the fall of 1995, Steven Schroeder, Nancy Kaufman, and Bill Novelli approached John Seffrin, chief executive officer of the American Cancer Society, about partnering with The Robert Wood Johnson Foundation in underwriting the National Center for Tobacco-Free Kids. Seffrin supported the concept, and got the approval of the Cancer Society's board for a financial commitment of $10 million over a five-year period. Buoyed by the presence of a solid financial and political partner, in January 1996, The Robert Wood Johnson Foundation authorized a grant of $20 million to support the National Center for Tobacco-Free Kids. (In 1999, the Foundation renewed and augmented its grant to the Center, awarding it $50 million for the period from April 1999 through March 2004.)

The Center originally had four objectives:

1. To develop a national strategy for reducing youth tobacco use
2. To serve as a media center that would develop national information efforts to prevent youth tobacco use and counter the promotional efforts of the tobacco industry

3. To provide intensive technical assistance to state and community public education efforts to improve their effectiveness

4. To broaden the base and the depth of national organizational support to reduce youth tobacco use.[5]

Given the nature of the Center's work, the Foundation re-emphasized that its funds could not be used for lobbying purposes.[6]

Those who had been active in the Coalition on Smoking OR Health were most affected by creation of the Center for Tobacco-Free Kids. Part of Matt Myers' responsibility was to soothe the ruffled feathers, especially among members of the Coalition, and to get the public health community to support the big new kid on the block in the antismoking movement.

Keeping peace and harmony within the public health community was essential, since all hands would be needed on deck to build public support for the FDA in its decision to assert jurisdiction over tobacco. Toward that end, one of the first objectives of Tobacco-Free Kids was to ratchet the anti-tobacco/pro-FDA activity level upward across the board, both in Washington and elsewhere.

As part of this effort, the Center for Tobacco-Free Kids began a series of discussions with public health organizations about why FDA jurisdiction over tobacco was important, and to prepare them to become public spokespersons about the question. It also began working with the American Heart Association, the American Cancer Society, the American Lung Association, the American Medical Association, and the American Academy of Pediatrics on the stand-and-be-counted issue of getting pledges of support from elected officials for the FDA's decision. "It was anticipated that the tobacco industry would go into Congress to try to cut off the FDA before it could ever move forward," Myers says. "Our goal was to beat them to the punch—to build as visible and as broad a base of support as possible that would send a signal to opponents that they would fail if they tried to kill it."

For a fledgling organization, coordinating all these activities in its first year of existence meant that Novelli, Myers, and the rest of the staff had to hit the ground running. Even so, they soon had to pick up the pace. While the issue of FDA jurisdiction over tobacco started working its way through Congress, a number of states had filed suit against the tobacco industry, seeking to recoup the cost of treating people who had developed cancer, emphysema, and other diseases as a result of smoking. Several litigating states had entered clandestine preliminary conversations with the Liggett group, one of the smaller tobacco companies—discussions that were expected to lead ultimately to a financial settlement. Early in 1996, a number of the state attorneys general approached Myers about opening channels of communication with the public health community.[7] As Myers recalls:

> The attorneys general secretly came to me to say they were pretty close to an agreement. They thought it was important to have the public health community see their settlement as a victory, and asked to me to review the agreement, and to act as a liaison—which I did. From that time on, I was in regular contact and communication with the state attorneys general, so that when they began a second round of negotiations with Liggett, they asked us to participate with them—which I did. That was not particularly controversial, but it was an important period when the relationship with the AGs developed very closely.

At about the same time, a number of the state attorneys general began a very tentative dialogue with other corporations in the tobacco industry, and with the White House, about the possibility of a much broader agreement, and with it a much heftier financial settlement. "When we got wind of that, we went into the White House to warn them about sham deals, which has been the history of tobacco industry settlements in the past, and to make clear to the White House that the public health community intended to scrutinize any agreements very closely," Myers says. "Bruce Lindsey, special assistant to the president, and I talked on a regular basis."

In March 1997, representatives of the tobacco industry approached the attorneys general and indicated that they had a very serious offer they wanted to put on the table. Concurrently, they communicated their intentions to the White House, which told them to call the National Center for Tobacco-Free Kids, and insisted that the organization had to be part of any discussions that would take place. Things moved quickly from then on, and from April 3 through June 20, 1997, Myers was an active participant in negotiations between the state attorneys general and Big Tobacco. For the first two weeks, those negotiations took place entirely in secret. On April 16, however, the *Wall Street Journal* broke the story that the talks were going on.[8] The revelation generated both widespread news coverage and a firestorm within the public health community.

The more militant antismoking activists felt that they had been sold down the river. Believing themselves betrayed, they were outraged by the idea that discussions were occurring at all: for them, it was an article of faith that one did not negotiate with the tobacco industry, any more than one would bargain with the Devil himself. Stanton Glantz, a professor at the University of California, San Francisco and founder of Americans for Non-Smokers Rights, argued, "In negotiating with the industry, Matt Myers chose to ignore a consensus among public health groups not to enter a deal with the industry. . . . Participation in the decision-making process has been kept to a small circle; history shows that broader involvement serves the public health."[9] Further, he felt that "the tobacco-control community now has a real opportunity to end the tobacco industry in this country. If that opportunity is lost, it will be because the National Center for Tobacco-Free Kids lost it for us."[10]

Rep. Henry Waxman (Democrat of California), another who had staunchly opposed the tobacco industry for many years, was upset at Myers's attempting to negotiate legislation with the industry. "I was critical of Matt Myers and whoever else was in there. They didn't coordinate with their colleagues in the advocacy world; they didn't coordinate with their allies on the Hill."[11]

From the outset, however, there was an inner circle within the public health community that was clued into the discussions. As a result of the prior settlement discussions between the attorneys general and the Liggett Group, Myers and Novelli had come to believe that further dialogue with the tobacco industry was in the offing even before the first overtures from Big Tobacco were made, and they had determined to prepare for that eventuality. In fact, even before negotiations with the tobacco industry as a whole had begun, Myers and several others had called together public health advocates to discuss the possibility that there would eventually be some form of compromise agreement offered. "We expected that the tobacco industry would make an offer secretly to the White House or to Congress, and we told our colleagues that we believed it was important that there be a discussion of what the public health community wanted out of any proposals," says Myers. However, the public health community could not, even at that early stage, agree upon goals and strategies. "It was our frustration at our inability to generate a broad, more public dialogue that led Bill Novelli and me to convene the leaders of the major public health organizations in private to begin to discuss these issues."

Beginning in January, 1997, and extending all the way through the negotiation period, Bill Novelli and Matt Myers conferred with an informal executive group that included the CEOs of the American Cancer Society, the American Heart Association, and the American Lung Association; the highest ranking representative of the Academy of Pediatrics; and a past president of the American Medical Association.

With this all-star kitchen cabinet as a sounding board, Novelli and Myers began gaming mock negotiation scenarios a full four months before discussions actually got under way in April. "They all had the opportunity to think through choices, to take a look at what they were willing to give up, what they weren't willing to give up," Myers says. Once the talks began, "the group got regular briefings, even before the negotiations became public knowledge. Bill and I set up conference calls with them every couple of days, in which I briefed them about what was being discussed and what the issues were."

As Novelli recalls:

> Matt and I talked every night, and we'd discuss how to make the deal better. Can we add something on smoking in the workplace, or smoking in public places? We were also keeping our allies—John Seffrin at the American Cancer Society; Dudley Hafner, CEO of the American Heart Association; Lonnie Bristow, past president of the American Medical Association; and John Garrison, CEO of the American Lung Association—abreast of what was going on. We didn't tell our staff. We felt that the negotiations had to be essentially secret. Once they became public, it was a bonfire.

"Sound and fury, light and anger, vitriol, nervousness—it was probably the most trying time the Center ever had," Myers says. "While the negotiations were going on, I made little more than token appearances at the office. A huge burden fell to Bill to manage the uproar and to manage the public response."

After the negotiations became public knowledge, discussions continued to take place, and progress continued to be made.With great fanfare the agreement was announced on June 20, 1997. It required the tobacco industry to make annual payments estimated to total $368.5 billion in the first 25 years and to continue indefinitely. "The settlement was signed by all of the attorneys general, but not by us," Myers says. "We took the position that it wasn't for us to sign or not sign. We were there as advisers, not parties."

Tobacco control provisions in the deal included:

- Full FDA authority over tobacco, including the power to curtail tobacco marketing and to reduce and/or eliminate harmful ingredients and components, including nicotine

- Significant curtailment of tobacco marketing, that included but exceeded restrictions proposed by the FDA in 1996

- A ban on all outdoor and Internet advertising

- The elimination of all human images and cartoon characters in tobacco ads

- Restrictions on point of sale advertising and vending machines

- A ban on all brand name sponsorship, the use of tobacco brand names on nontobacco items, like hats and t-shirts, and a ban on free giveaways of nontobacco items based on the purchase of tobacco products

- Severe limits on tobacco ads in magazines with large youth readership

- Nationwide restrictions on youth access to tobacco products

- The adoption of tougher more visible new health warnings on packs and ads

- Nationwide standards to curtail exposure to secondhand smoke

- Penalties of up to $2 billion a year if youth smoking rates did not fall by 50% in 7 years and 60% in 10 years

- $1.5 billion a year to be used for tobacco cessation and $1 billion a year for tobacco-prevention efforts

In exchange, the companies won freedom from class action lawsuits and from the award of punitive damages based on prior acts by tobacco manufacturers, as well as a $5 billion annual ceiling on the total amount of damages the tobacco industry would be required to pay to successful litigants.

After the terms of the settlement were announced, the National Center for Tobacco-Free Kids and Myers personally became targets of opportunity for outraged anti-tobacco activists who had opposed the discussions, and for those who believed the settlement to be a sellout of the public interest. "The fact that we had, even before it became public, asked the other public health organizations if they would like to participate, and urged several of them to do so, didn't make an awful lot of difference to outsiders," Myers says. Among the most vocal opponents of the settlement were Rep. Henry Waxman, outgoing FDA chief Kessler, former Surgeon General Koop, and consumer advocate Ralph Nader.

"The National Center for Tobacco-Free Kids is performing exactly the wrong role," said Waxman, a longtime tobacco foe. "They seem to have forgotten that their original mission was to be advocates, not back-room negotiators."[12]

Nader wrote to Myers and his colleagues:

A disturbing transformation is discernible in the approach of the public health advocates who have been involved in the litigation settlement negotiations. . . . While they originally promised only to support an exploration of the negotiation option, they have now become active proponents of a settlement deal. . . . This premature support for a settlement suggests that those involved in the negotiations and their close supporters have become invested in the negotiation process, and that this has distorted their ability to evaluate clearly the costs and benefits of a deal. At a minimum, the venality and historic duplicity of the tobacco industry are sufficient for any public health advocate not to lend credence to any tobacco industry deal that immunizes it from the only branch of government whose processes they could not buy or rent—the judiciary.[13]

A committee to review the settlement, organized by Waxman and chaired by Koop and Kessler, condemned the settlement. Even Dudley Hafner of the American Heart Association denounced the plan as "totally unacceptable." "These provisions have been very well lawyered by the tobacco industry to thwart gains already made," Kessler told reporters after the settlement was announced. "It's giving away the farm."[14]

The fate of "the farm" did not, of course, rest solely, or even primarily, with the Center for Tobacco-Free Kids. The various attorneys general who were plaintiffs in the lawsuits had the most to say about the final terms of settlement. Significantly, however, who those AGs were, and how many there were, changed as negotiations went on. At the outset, the small cadre of participating attorneys general shared a common belief that the tobacco industry should reimburse the states for the health care costs they had incurred and were likely to incur in the future. Between April and June, however, the number of states that were suing the tobacco companies grew geometrically, if only because nobody wanted to be left off the gravy train. What happened, according to Myers, is that

> the state attorneys general who cared about the public health issues dominated those discussions and the results reflected their concerns. The new state attorneys general who became involved, however, were so anxious to reach an agreement that they undermined any opposition to the provisions granting the tobacco industry relief from class actions and punitive damages.

The state attorneys general had been promised by the White House, which had monitored the negotiations closely, that President Clinton would declare his support for the settlement within twenty-four hours of its public announcement. Myers was not surprised when several days, weeks, and even months later, the AGs were still waiting. "As the one Washington person in the group, I kept saying to the AGs, 'You guys are pretty sophisticated, but if you believe that one, I've got a bridge to sell you.' And in fact what the White House did was to step back and say, 'I'm going to wait and see which way the wind is blowing. And you guys who I pushed out on this limb—you sort of stay out there awhile. When there's a consensus, we'll be right there to support you.' " [15]

—⁂— In Congress: The McCain Bill

The June 20 settlement needed federal legislation to become effective, and the Republican leadership of the Senate sent the matter to the Commerce Committee, chaired by John McCain, Republican of Arizona. Although until that time McCain had never evinced much interest in the subject of tobacco, he now took the issue seriously and asked for help from the National Center for Tobacco-Free Kids in drafting legislation that would implement the agreement between the AGs and the tobacco companies. "We'd already developed a relationship with him," Myers says. "He came to us saying, 'I'm going to start holding hearings. I want to explore this issue, and it would be my goal to introduce a bill that the whole public health community could endorse, and I don't intend to consult with the tobacco industry about what ought to be in it.' "

Myers worked with McCain's office to put a bill together.[16] Introduced in March 1998, it breezed through the Commerce Committee in April by a vote of nineteen to one—but without the endorsement of the public health community. Not only that, but Koop and Kessler strongly opposed enacting the terms of the settlement into legislation. Koop testified before the Commerce Committee that "The settlement gives the tobacco industry everything it wants, but short-changes the public health."

Myers says:

> I believe that not supporting the bill is one of the most serious mistakes the public health community has ever made. It was truly the most far-reaching anti-tobacco bill that's ever been considered in this country. Both David Kessler and C. Everett Koop decided that the bill still wasn't good enough. Had the public health community endorsed the bill at that point, it probably would have flown to the floor of the Senate and passed with eighty votes. As it was, however, because the public health community was divided, Trent Lott announced that he thought the Senate needed more time to study the issue.

What happened after that proved once more that politics makes strange bedfellows. Progressive Democrats introduced amendments to put more teeth in the law, and were supported not only by their liberal confreres but by arch conservatives as well—though for diametrically opposite reasons. The former group was trying to strengthen the bill, but the latter was trying to turn it into a "Christmas tree," festooned with riders and provisos ensuring that it would never pass.

Lott, the Senate majority leader, put the bill on hold for six weeks, a delay that allowed the tobacco industry to conduct their TV advertising against the bill. The bill was then on the floor of the Senate for a full month, the longest that any piece of proposed legislation had been on the Senate floor since the days of the civil rights movement, and long enough for the tobacco manufactureres to go after McCain's bill with a vengeance. They threw all of their considerable advertising, political, and financial resources into the battle. The tobacco industry announced its opposition, launched a $40 million TV advertising campaign criticizing the bill as pork-barrel legislation, and then spent $60 million more lobbying against the bill.

Despite Big Tobacco's big guns, Bill Novelli still believed that the anti-smoking forces would carry the day. "The tobacco industry basically said, 'The public health community can't be trusted. The Senate has loaded up this bill, and the provisions are far too onerous. Not only are we walking away from this legislation, we're going to kill it.' When that happened, I said to myself, 'They can't win this. They're going to go to the people; they're going to put up a huge advertising campaign, and it's going to be a bust, because nobody is going to believe the tobacco industry . . .'—and I was wrong." On June 17, nearly a year to the day after the original settlement was first announced, the fate of McCain's bill came down to a vote on the Senate floor over a filibuster. "A total of fifty-seven senators—out of the sixty we needed—voted in favor of breaking it," Myers recalls sadly, "and forty-two voted against, which meant the bill died—and with it the opportunity to make a giant leap forward in tobacco control."

"The only thing I think I might have done differently," Novelli says, "would have been to go back to Steve Schroeder at The Robert Wood Johnson Foundation and say, 'Steve, I need another $50 million right now.' If we had been able to fight them dollar for dollar, or at least close to it, we might have been able to apply enough pressure to negate their message and to force the legislation through. Everything else I think we did as best we could, with as much courage as we had, and as many resources as we had."

The failure to pass enabling legislation at the federal level put the state attorneys general back to square one. Because most of them had never intended to take their lawsuits to trial, they still needed to strike a bargain with the tobacco companies. Unfortunately, this was no secret. Just two weeks after the downfall of the McCain bill, confidential negotiations resumed, this time without any representatives from the public health community at the table. Although Myers maintained his back door communication with those AGs who had been part of the original group of litigants, everyone knew they were negotiating in a distinctly different political landscape. "The folks who were our friends had limited power," he says. "There were four or five who had always believed in what they did, and really wanted to get the best deal for the public that they could, but they didn't have a lot of leverage, because everybody knew that the threat of going to trial wasn't real. The vast majority of the AGs who had suits pending had only one question: how much do I get and when do I get it?" At the end of the day, what had started as a public health issue had come down to getting Big Tobacco to "show me the money," in the *Jerry Maguire* catchphrase of the moment.

—⟋⟍— After the Defeat of the McCain Bill

The demise of the McCain bill marked the beginning of a new chapter for the Center for Tobacco-Free Kids as well. Of necessity, this phase began with an embrace of the inevitable—the acceptance that there would be another, and probably weaker settlement between the attorneys general and the tobacco industry.

At what might understandably have been considered a dark hour, the staff rallied and dug in for a long, hard slog in the trenches. "Even while Congress was turning away from tobacco, the level of energy out of this office was ramping up, not down," Myers says. Because of the urgency involved in dealing with the FDA issue, the state attorneys general lawsuit and the McCain bill, one of the Center's original objectives—to provide intensive technical assistance to state and community efforts—had to this point been secondary to efforts at the federal level. Now, however, it took center stage.

The time had come to sharpen the skills of local antismoking activists—to work with them to hone their marketing and public relations skills. "I call it 'professionalizing the movement,'" the Foundation's Joe Marx says. "The people involved with tobacco control had the passion and had been fighting the good fight for years and years, but needed the kind of savvy, innovation, and creativity that Bill Novelli brought with him."

Novelli and Myers brought in outside professionals—it didn't matter whether they knew anything about tobacco and about the tobacco industry; they knew how to create advertising messages that had an impact on people. Today the Center maintains advisers and an inventory of supplies that can equip and energize antismoking activists in all fifty states with data, game plans, and communications materials.

Over the summer and the fall of 1998, the Center began mobilizing state by state. "We immediately got out talking points to public health advocates all over the country," Myers says. "With funding from The Robert Wood Johnson

Foundation, we organized a conference in which we brought together tobacco control advocates from every state. We prepared briefing materials for them, to arm them to return home and begin working for the use of settlement money for tobacco prevention." On November 23, 1998, the attorneys general for 46 states[17] and the tobacco industry announced the completion of another agreement. The Master Settlement Agreement[18] includes the following provisions:

- Elimination of most but not all outdoor advertising
- Termination of cartoon images in marketing—Joe Camel was gone, but the Marlboro man lives on
- Dissolution of the Tobacco Institute, the Council on Tobacco Research, and the Center for Indoor Air Research
- Prohibition of youth targeting in marketing
- Prohibition of product placement in films and television
- Curtailment of vending machines to adults-only facilities

Matt Myers comments that the Master Settlement Agreement was far weaker and narrower than either the June 1997 agreement or the McCain legislation. "It did not provide the FDA with authority over tobacco. It did not penalize tobacco companies if youth smoking rates did not decline. It did not set standards for protection against secondhand smoke. It did not strengthen or revise health warnings on tobacco products or ads. There was nothing in the agreement that required retailers be licensed, that ingredients in tobacco products be disclosed or that harmful ingredients in tobacco products be removed. It did not require that any money be used for tobacco prevention or cessation, and the $300 million a year that was provided to the American Legacy Foundation for five years had restrictions on it."

By the time the Master Settlement Agreement was announced, local activists were ready to rumble. The National Center for Tobacco-Free Kids had already laid the groundwork to do battle in every state in the union and had prioritized about twenty states to be the focus of legislative action. "We produced state-specific data, so that representatives from every state would have fact sheets indicating the number of smokers, how much the tobacco industry spends, and how much the state spends on health care to deal with smoking-related illnesses," Myers says. "They didn't have to reinvent that wheel every time they needed information."

Once the settlement was announced, one of the functions of the Center was to keep antismoking advocates abreast of what their fellow activists were doing. Among the innovations that evolved during this period was use of the Internet for exchanging information and ideas among tobacco control activists. People in Ohio could compare notes with advocates in Washington or Rhode Island. The communication was both informative and energizing. "When bills with identical language popped up in four different states, we could generally figure out that they had been written by someone from a tobacco company, because we knew from talking to one another that it wasn't just a coincidence when this suddenly started happening," Myers says. "I think it was the first time that individuals in various states who are fighting these battles didn't perceive themselves as isolated islands, but, rather, as part of a national network."

The Center for Tobacco-Free Kids also put its Washington-based advertising expertise in service to local and state antismoking activists. "We had our agency create flexible model ads that could be used in a number of ways," Myers says. "If an ad fit a theme in a given state, advocates could simply drop in the names and figures as needed. They didn't have to incur any creative costs at all; all they needed to do to run the ad was to buy space or time. It was a huge financial bonus."

—∿— Learning How to Do It

Since the settlement, the Center for Tobacco-Free Kids has pushed a broad agenda designed to increase funding for tobacco prevention and cessation, to protect against second-hand smoke, and to increase state taxes on tobacco products. It has also worked to deveop nationwide support for providing the FDA with jurisdiction over tobacco. As the battleground shifted to the states, the professionalization of the movement began to pay off. "We've learned how to do it," Myers says. "Four years ago, Maine had the highest teenage smoking rate in the nation, over 39 percent. In four years, that number has gone down to 25 percent. Mississippi and Florida are right behind them—and both of them used settlement money to do it. There is no single magic bullet—we're dealing with a complex human behavior. The states that have succeeded have taken a multipronged, multifaceted approach, and that's what's critical—the combination of mass media advertising, funding for local community groups, and school-based programs. Taken together, they've been found to be more effective than enforcement of the laws against sales to minors."

"For too long we've found lung cancer rates to be an acceptable fact of life," Matt Myers says. "They're no more of an inevitability and necessity than polio. We're not used to funding tobacco prevention. If we saw it as the equivalent of a vaccine against lung cancer—and it is—then the money wouldn't be an issue. We can now say with a fair degree of scientific certainty that we know how to significantly reduce the incidence of tobacco use among kids. We do not yet know how to eliminate it, or to reduce it to a minimally acceptable level, but we do know how to dramatically impact it—and that's a start."

Notes

1. (http://rjrtdocs.com/rjrtdocs/image_viewer.dms?DOC_RANGE=502033156 +-3157&PS=4&GOTO=2&SEARCH=1382&CAMEFROM=3&SIZE=1)
2. Arkin, E. B. "Needs for Communication Support for the Denormalization of Tobacco Use." (Unpublished, 1994)
3. For a description of the Tobacco Institute, see "Inside PR." (www.reputation-mgmt.com/tobacco.htm)
4. Together with other tobacco-related organizations, including the Council for Tobacco Research and the Council for Indoor Air Research, the Tobacco Institute was dissolved by the November 1998 Master Settlement Agreement between the state attorneys general and the tobacco industry.
5. Since the inception of the Center, two additional objectives have been added: (1) build support for enactment of comprehensive national tobacco control legislation; and (2) increase relationships with tobacco growers, their communities, and their allies.

6. In a letter to the *New York Times* dated December 15, 1997, Bill Novelli wrote, "We do not employ foundation funds for lobbying."
7. Mississippi Attorney General Mike Moore filed suit in May 1994, asking for $940 million in damages. In March 1996, Liggett settled with five states, including Mississippi.
8. Freedman, A., and Hwang, S. "Peace Pipe: Philip Morris, RJR, and Tobacco Plaintiffs Discuss a Settlement." *Wall Street Journal,* Apr. 16, 1997.

    According to Matt Myers, the story was planted, but the manner in which word of the talks leaked to the press is unclear. Carrick Mollenkamp, Adam Levy, Joseph Menn, and Jeffrey Rothfeder of Bloomberg News, authors of *The People vs. Big Tobacco* (Princeton: Bloomberg Press, 1998), who covered the talks while they were in progress, say, "By Tuesday, April 15, Alix Freedman, a Wall Street Journal tobacco reporter . . . learned that Big Tobacco and its opponents had been meeting steadily for the past two weeks. Some speculate that the tip came from RJR, while others think the leak emanated from [Minnesota AG] Hubert Humphrey III, who was complaining that he wasn't given a big-enough role at the negotiating table. Both deny tipping Freedman off" (p. 142).

    There is no question, however, that tobacco industry stockholders profited significantly by the revelation that talks were ongoing. By the end of that trading day on Wall Street, shares of Philip Morris had "soared $4.13 to $43.13, up 11 percent, as more than 18 million shares changed hands. *That increased the value of the company's stock market worth by $10 billion—a one-day jump greater than the entire market value of Federal Express* (emphasis added). RJR's stock also shot up 11 percent, or $3.25. 'It was the best news for the industry since matches were invented,' said Marc Perkins, a money manager in Jupiter, Florida" (Mollenkamp, Levy, Menn, and Rothfeder, 1998, p. 144).
9. Pertschuk, M. *Smoke in Their Eyes: Lessons in Movement Leadership From the Tobacco Wars.* Nashville: Vanderbuilt University, 2001, p. 97.
10. Pertschuk (2001), p. 99.
11. Pertschuk (2001), p. 105.
12. Stolberg, S. G. "Beleaguered Tobacco Foe Holds Key to Talks." *New York Times,* June 4, 1997. (http://query.nytimes.com/search/restricted/article?res=F50C1EF738590C1EF738590C778CDDAF0894)
13. June 19, 1997, letter from Ralph Nader to Matthew Myers and others. (www.tobacco.org/News/970619nader.html)

14. Mollenkamp, Levy, Menn, and Rothfeder (1998), p. 238.

15. Despite the fact that Hugh Rodham (brother of Hillary Clinton) was at the bargaining table, the White House did not come forward on behalf of the settlement until September 17. On that date, "flanked by Mike Moore, C. Everett Koop, David Kessler, and Matt Myers, Clinton delivered his much anticipated verdict on the agreement. While he stopped short of a full endorsement, Clinton urged Congress to put the tobacco settlement into law" (Mollenkamp, et al., 1998, p. 244).

16. This assistance was provided using non-foundation funds. See note 7, op. cit.

17. Four states—Mississippi, Florida, Texas, and Minnesota—settled separately with the tobacco industry.

18. The complete text of the Master Settlement Agreement is available online from the National Association of Attorneys General (www.naag.org). A summary of its provisions can be found on the Website of the Office of the Attorney General of the State of California (http://caag.state.ca.us/tobacco/resources/msasumm.htm). For a table comparing provisions of the 1998 MSA with the original 1997 agreement and the McCain bill, see www.tobaccofreekids.org.

6

Helping Addicted Smokers Quit

The Foundation's Tobacco-Cessation Programs

C. Tracy Orleans and Joseph Alper

Editors' Introduction

The Robert Wood Johnson Foundation often supports research or demonstration projects to determine whether a specific type of intervention works—a new organizational strategy, an innovative financing method, an improved treatment. The thought behind this approach is that good ideas are picked up and spread widely. This does not always happen, however. Perhaps the research is convincing, but something more is needed before it gets translated into standard practice. Such is the case with tobacco cessation. The research clearly shows the benefits of certain approaches—those employing counseling and pharmaceuticals. These approaches don't even take much time. Yet they are not widely practiced by physicians or within health care organizations. This chapter examines the Foundation's efforts to translate research into practice to help smokers quit.

The long translation effort began with research to determine which interventions were effective. Once effective treatments were identified and formalized in federal guidelines issued in 1996, the Foundation sought to make them a regular part of medical practice. Its approach included publicizing the guidelines, using them as the basis of standards, attempting to create demand for them, and coaxing insurers to cover the cost of using them.

Much of the Foundation's work has been with managed care organizations. As organized delivery systems that can track patients and benefit from keeping people healthier, managed care organizations should have an incentive to offer a preventive service such as tobacco cessation. However, frequent turnover of enrollees from one plan to another obscures the financial benefits for any given managed care plan and has slowed adoption of tobacco-cessation treatments.

The Foundation's support of efforts to help people quit smoking illustrates the challenge of translating science into medical practice, the difficulty of overcoming addiction (even when people say they want to stop), and the need for a variety of approaches to speed adoption of what seems like a commonsense idea. It also highlights the tension between investment to prevent a problem and investment to treat a problem. To date, the Foundation has invested in both prevention and treatment; it devotes a majority of its antitobacco funding to keeping young people from starting to smoke, while still investing (though less significantly) in helping current smokers quit. Of course, smoking-cessation programs might be considered a form of secondary prevention. The chapter makes the disturbing point that every state Medicaid program covers expensive, intensive medical care to treat people with lung cancer but only twenty-four state Medicaid programs cover treatment to help smokers quit.

This chapter is written by C. Tracy Orleans, senior scientist at The Robert Wood Johnson Foundation, who has been a key player in developing the Foundation's smoking-cessation strategy; and Joseph Alper, an award-winning freelance writer who has contributed chapters to previous volumes of *The Robert Wood Johnson Foundation Anthology* series.

In a typical week, thirty-five thousand American teenagers try their first cigarette, and fourteen thousand become regular smokers, with more than half going on to a lifetime of nicotine addiction. Most of these smokers will try to quit their habit numerous times, some of them successfully, most not. A third of the teenagers who get hooked on cigarettes will die as a result.

Some forty years ago, Bob Clement[1] became a teenage smoker. Now fifty-four and living in a suburb of Seattle, Clement, a retired police officer, is a pack-a-day smoker whose only break from his tobacco addiction came during the four times he has tried to quit smoking cold turkey over the past fifteen or so years. Clement is a realist. He knows that smoking is damaging his health and will probably kill him eventually if he continues. He also knows how hard it will be to quit for more than the couple of months that he usually lasts before picking up a pack of cigarettes at his local gas station. But this time, he says, he has an added incentive: "Hunting season is coming, and smoking has finally gotten me to the point where I get winded so easily I won't be able to follow my prey. That is completely unacceptable."

This extra motivation has prompted him to take what for him is a radical step: getting help. "I've tried quitting on my own, and I guess I can't do it," says Clement with a grave laugh. "What can you do to help me?"

Kathy Nago, who is talking on the phone with Clement, hears this plea a dozen times a day. She is one of seventy trained smoking-cessation counselors answering the phones at the Tukwila, Washington, facility of Group Health Cooperative of Puget Sound. This is a routing place for smokers who call in on one of the toll-free "quit lines" sponsored by Washington, Oregon, Minnesota, Wisconsin, Maine, Utah, and Georgia for the citizens of each state, as well as one for all Group Health Cooperative members. On this beautiful fall morning, Nago has already given advice to a shy fortysomething woman from Oregon who was making her first attempt to quit, and has transferred a call from a thirty-nine-year-old Minnesota smoker to a counselor at HealthPartners, a managed care company in the Minneapolis-St. Paul area that runs its own quit line.

Nago's first task with Clement is to engage him in friendly conversation while gathering some general background information—age, address, insurance company, and the like—and baseline information about his smoking habits, his overall health, and his previous attempts to quit. She is particularly interested in the hows and whys of his previous attempts and in his current motivation to quit, entering all of this information into an online database that will be available to every other counselor if Clement calls back later for further help. She finds out he has never used a nicotine replacement product, such as nicotine gum or a controlled-release patch; when she informs him that nicotine replacement therapy doubles the success rate of quitting, she can hear from the way he says, "Really? How do I get some?" that she has hit the right button.

Given Clement's smoking habits, Nago recommends that he start with an over-the-counter nicotine patch at a strength of 21 milligrams. While she's telling him how to use the patch, she browses the information on her computer screen and finds that Clement's insurance covers over-the-counter nicotine replacement therapy and will also cover the cost of limited-duration group counseling. He's not interested in "that touchy-feely stuff," he says, but he is interested in receiving any written materials that might help because, as he says, "I'm a good learner when I can read something."

From her computer terminal, Nago orders a videotape and a collection of materials (tailored to his age and to the fact that he has tried to quit before) to be sent to Clement. Then, in a final, all-important step, Nago gets Clement to commit to a specific date to quit. "How about this Friday?" he says.

"Can you get to the store and have nicotine patches by then?"

"Absolutely," he responds. "Can you have the reading materials to me by then?"

Nago smiles. "I think you're going to do great this time," she says, "but make sure you call again if you have any concerns or start running into trouble. It's always free to call, and we're always here to help."

—〰— A Struggle Against Death and Disease

Armed with the nicotine patch, help from the Washington Quit Line, strong motivation, and insights gained from past attempts to quit, Clement stands a far-better-than-average chance of joining the forty-four million other Americans who call themselves former smokers.

Tobacco use and addiction are the nation's most important cause of preventable disease and premature death. More than 25 percent of adults and more than 30 percent of high school seniors, nearly fifty million Americans in total, report regular tobacco use. The consequences are staggering. Tobacco use and dependence are responsible for more than 430,000 premature deaths—approximately one in five deaths—every year. Heart disease, stroke, lung disease, cancer, and other chronic illnesses all result from regular smoking. Maternal smoking in pregnancy is the most important preventable cause of low birth weight, mortality in newborns, and sudden infant death syndrome.

The estimated cost to the American health care system is $80 billion in direct expenditures and $50 billion in indirect costs.[2] "The single biggest impact we could have on both the overall health of Americans and on reducing the escalating costs of health care would be to convert far more smokers into ex-smokers," says Dr. Michael Fiore, director of the Center for Tobacco Research and Intervention at the University of Wisconsin Medical School in Madison. "And while it's critically important that we work hard to prevent more Americans from becoming smokers, the greatest reductions in preventable mortality, morbidity, and health care burden over the next thirty to forty years will come from helping people quit smoking."

Although the prevalence of smoking has dropped by almost 40 percent since the Surgeon General's report on tobacco in 1964, more than half of all Americans who have ever smoked still smoke. Perhaps more indicative of how poorly we, as a nation, do in helping smokers quit their habit is the fact that though more than two-thirds of smokers say they want to quit, and half of them make at least one serious attempt to quit in any given year, only 2.5 percent—about 1.2 million a year—are able to quit smoking permanently.[3] "It's tragic—pathetic, really—that we do so poorly at helping people quit smoking," says Jack Hollis, associate director of the Kaiser Permanente Center for Health Research. "Particularly since we have smoking-cessation methods at our disposal that work and could have a much bigger impact if we could only get smokers to use them."

—ɯ— The Gap Between What We Know and What We Do

Nearly two decades of research and development have generated a wealth of phar-macological and behavioral tools that can effectively treat what is essentially a chronic disease, namely, nicotine addiction. Indeed, the U.S. Public Health Service issued clinical practice guidelines in 1996 and 2000 identifying a variety of treat-ments that could reduce tobacco-related disease and death dramatically. Through use of these treatments, the proportion of adult smokers who achieve long-term success when trying to quit on their own can be increased from 7 percent to as high as 30 percent.[4] Providing these treatments, including brief minimal-contact approaches designed to be integrated into everyday clinical practice, to the 70 percent of adult smokers who see their providers every year would double our national annual rate of quitting.

Such interventions are underused, however, reaching less than a quar-ter of all smokers. Summarizing this state of affairs, the Public Health Service, in *Treating Tobacco Use and Dependence: A Clinical Practice Guideline,* said, "It is difficult to identify a condition in the United States that presents such a mix of lethality, prevalence, and neglect, and for which effective interventions are so readily available."[5] As Susan Curry, director of the Health Research and Policy Centers at the University of Illinois at Chicago, puts it, "It's as if the medical pro-fession decided to ignore diabetes and high blood pressure, which, like cigarette smoking, are chronic diseases that are associated with so-called lifestyle deci-sions on the part of the individual, and for which the long-term treatment suc-cess rates are similar."

Tobacco researchers talk about the gap between what we know and what we do. What we know is that most smokers want to quit, most see a doctor at least once a year, and most doctors want to help them quit. Moreover, we know that the nation could double its current national annual rate of quitting if doctors routinely offered brief advice, counseling, and effective pharmacotherapy (such as the nico-tine patch or Zyban) that the *Guideline* recommends. Unfortunately, only 50–60 percent of smokers report getting any advice on quitting from their physicians, and fewer than 25 percent report any further counseling or drug-based therapy. Low-income and minority smokers are the least likely to get this help.

Granted, the gap between what we know and what we do has grown smaller. The number of quitters who currently make use of effective treatments is somewhere between 20 and 30 percent, which is twice as high as it was a decade ago.[6] There are plenty of reasons to explain why this gap has not shrunk further:

- Doctors and other primary care practitioners are not trained to deliver tobacco-cessation therapies. For example, fewer than 20 percent of medical schools offer even three hours of clinical instruction in treating tobacco addiction.[7]

- Physicians underestimate the difficulty smokers face in overcoming tobacco addiction and feel discouraged by what they perceive as their own lack of success in helping them. Even those who qualify (by helping their patients quit) for what Fiore calls "the good doctor club" note that if they succeed in getting one in five of their smoking patients to stop—a major public health achievement—results are typically delayed and invisible.

- The health care system does not support tobacco-cessation efforts. Surveys funded by The Robert Wood Johnson Foundation show that physicians who work to put the clinical practice *Guideline* into action do so without reminder and follow-up systems, without access to self-help materials, telephone quit lines, or community programs required to deliver effective counseling outside the eighteen-minute clinical visit.

- Insurance coverage and reimbursement policies often do not cover tobacco-dependence treatment that is known to be effective. Medicare, for example, still provides no coverage, and in 2000 only thirty-three states provided Medicaid coverage for any of the proven treatments recommended by the *Guideline*.

- The business case for tobacco-dependence treatment has not been made. Most purchasers of health care (such as large corporations), most policy makers, and most benefit consultants are not aware of the actual costs of illness related to smoking or of the economic benefits of quitting.[8] Businesses are unenthusiastic about anything but an immediate return on investment. "Health plans are fighting for their financial lives right now, and many of them claim that since member turnover is so high, they won't realize the savings three or four years down the road for money they're spending today," says Barbara Lardy, director of medical affairs for the American Association of Health Plans, managed care's national trade organization.

■ The community treating tobacco dependence does not think along policy lines. During a time when prevention policies were driving down the number of young people who took up smoking, few advocates focused on the power of these policies to induce smokers to quit. Similarly, until recently, policy makers and policy researchers largely ignored policy and regulatory strategies for tobacco cessation.

■ Even though most smokers want to quit and try to do so, this desire has not translated into demand for treatment. In a focus group funded by The Robert Wood Johnson Foundation, officials from health plans offering the most generous smoking-cessation treatments and benefits voiced a common frustration over smokers' generally low use of these services.[9] Not that there has been much done to build demand. Aside from recent direct-to-consumer advertising for nicotine gum and patches and Zyban, there have been few efforts to educate smokers about effective treatment. Aids and programs to reduce tobacco dependence are far less available to smokers than are cigarettes.

—ɯ— Closing the Gap: Foundation Goals and Strategies

In 1991, The Robert Wood Johnson Foundation adopted its current goal of reducing the harm caused by tobacco, alcohol, and illicit drugs. For tobacco, keeping children and teens from becoming smokers was the top priority. But the Foundation staff also saw a need to help addicted smokers quit. In both prevention and cessation, the staff sought to build on and complement the efforts of other tobacco-control funders, to finance initiatives that others could not, and to fill critical gaps.

The Foundation found two ways to further cessation efforts: first, by identifying and promoting effective tobacco-cessation treatments; and second, by translating research on successful treatment into practice. It focused its grants and programs on three underserved and important populations—pregnant smokers, managed care enrollees, and adolescents—and, as shown in Figure 6.1, adopted a three-pronged approach to reach these populations:

1. Improving the scientific basis for and the knowledge of effective tobacco-dependence treatment

2. Building the capacity of health care systems to deliver effective intervention

3. Building a market and demand (among health care providers, purchasers, policy makers, and consumers) for them

—ⱳ— Improving the Scientific Basis for and Knowledge of Effective Treatment

The Foundation's efforts have focused on developing and disseminating federal guidelines to aid physicians and other health care professionals in delivering tobacco-cessation treatment. The guidelines examine the relevant research and make recommendations about the kinds of tobacco-cessation intervention that have been shown to be effective.

In 1996, the federal Agency for Health Care Policy and Research, or AHCPR (since renamed the Agency for Healthcare Research and Quality), created an expert panel to review the scientific literature on smoking cessation and to identify treatments that worked. This review culminated with publication of the federal government's first clinical practice *Guideline*. It recommended an intervention of three to five minutes that physicians, nurses, dentists, and smoking-cessation specialists could deliver during a routine primary care visit. It also defined effective behavioral counseling methods and pharmacotherapies.

Once the first guideline was issued, The Robert Wood Johnson Foundation collaborated with the AHCPR and other funders in organizing a national conference in Washington, D.C., to let key provider organizations, policy makers, and tobacco-control advocates know about the *Guideline* and how it could be used to expand the benefits offered by Medicare, Medicaid, managed care plans, and private insurance companies.

Figure 6.1   Getting Evidence-based Tobacco Treatments into Practice

Goal
To increase the adoption, reach, and impact of
evidence-based tobacco-dependence treatments

Improving the scientific basis for and the knowledge of effective tobacco-dependence treatments	**Building the capacity of health care systems to deliver effective tobacco-dependence treatments**	**Creating demand for effective tobacco-dependence treatments**
■ Formal clinical practice guidelines	■ Provider training and implementation tools	■ Accreditation and performance measurement
■ Test and adapt interventions in new populations or settings	■ Technical assistance for "real world" practice settings	■ Increased coverage and reimbursement
■ Research and develop more effective and feasible interventions	■ Systems-level changes, such as information and reminder systems to identify smokers and cue providers, performance feedback systems, and incentive programs	■ Making the business case
		■ Direct-to-consumer market research and marketing

Increase the number of:
- ■ practitioners providing evidence-based tobacco-dependence treatments
- ■ systems providing evidence-based tobacco-dependence treatments
- ■ individuals receiving evidence-based tobacco-dependence treatments

Ultimate Goal
To reduce tobacco use and tobacco-caused disease and health care burden

The Foundation also awarded a series of grants to organizations and professional societies having a strong track record in educating health care providers and setting national practice standards. Grantees included the American Medical Association, the American Nurses Foundation, the American College of Obstetricians and Gynecologists, the American Women's Medical Association, and the American Academy of Pediatrics.

These organizations publicized the *Guideline* through their professional journals and meetings and developed aids for special populations, such as pregnant smokers, teenage smokers, and smokers in low-income and minority populations. "We knew that professional society endorsement was critical to providers' adopting previous clinical practice guidelines, but we also learned from the professional societies that the *Guideline* alone wasn't enough," said Harriet Bennett, the tobacco liaison for the Agency for Healthcare Research and Quality, who oversaw the agency's efforts to disseminate the *Guideline*. "They needed more tailored information and more practical tools, like pocket reminders and patient handouts." One such tool that the Foundation helped to fund and disseminate was a short parallel guideline from the AHCPR on the health care system changes (such as adding a tobacco user identification system and including tobacco-dependence treatment as a covered benefit) that were required to fully integrate *Guideline*-based care into routine clinical practice.

Given rapid growth in the scientific evidence, the U.S. Public Health Service reconvened the original expert panel, which reviewed three thousand more articles published between 1995 and 1999 and issued an updated *Guideline* in 2000. The new *Guideline* recommended a brief primary care intervention, now known as the 5-As, which had been demonstrated to be effective in getting smokers to quit:

1. *Ask* every patient about tobacco use and smoking.
2. *Advise* all smokers to quit.
3. *Assess* smokers' willingness to quit.
4. *Assist* those who are motivated with brief counseling, self-help materials, and pharmacotherapy (nicotine replacement products and Zyban) and those who are not with brief motivational counseling.
5. *Arrange* follow-up for continued support and more intensive treatment if needed.

The 5-A model requires as little as two minutes of a physician's time. This may not seem like much, but research has demonstrated that if a physician with no special training in behavioral counseling spends only two minutes advising patients to quit smoking, twice as many quit as would do so without even this briefest of interventions.[10] By itself, this would produce an additional 1.2 million former smokers annually—slightly more than the number of individuals who become smokers each year.

The *Guideline* endorsed a team approach, making it clear that the entire burden of smoking cessation is not meant to fall on the shoulders of primary care physicians. "I'm a practicing primary care physician, and I can tell you that it's hard to think about adding another two-minute task into the already crowded ten to fifteen minutes that I get for a routine office visit," says Charles J. Bentz, medical co-director of the smoking cessation and prevention effort for Providence Health System's Portland Oregon region. "That's why it's so important that we make this a systems approach involving every member of the team."

Michael Fiore, who served as panel chairman for the original and updated *Guideline,* agrees that the 5-A model calls for a team approach: "It starts from the time a patient walks through the door and encounters the receptionist and continues all the way to when a patient picks up a prescription for nicotine replacement therapy or Zyban from the pharmacist and talks with a telephone quit-line counselor for additional counseling and support." This team extends to counselors outside the primary care context. Confirming a strong relationship between the intensity of tobacco-dependence counseling and its effectiveness, the *Guideline* recommends more intensive person-to-person counseling, particularly from experienced tobacco-dependence treatment specialists for smokers needing more help.

In addition to providing funds to update the *Guideline,* the Foundation contributed again to efforts to communicate and implement it. In 2000, it joined the Agency for Healthcare Research and Quality, the American Cancer Society, the Centers for Disease Control and Prevention, and the National Cancer Institute to support development of a plan for putting the *Guideline* into practice. In collaboration with the American Cancer Society, the Foundation also co-funded a new national Cessation Treatment Center, based in Washington, D.C., to guide, monitor, and stimulate efforts to implement the plan.

The Foundation has paid particular attention to developing and disseminating recommendations for pregnant smokers, investing approximately $25 million over the past ten years in Smoke-Free Families. The program, whose goal is to eliminate smoking during and beyond pregnancy, funds both a National Program Office to support research on treatment innovations and a National Dissemination Office to promote widespread adoption of existing best practices. To assist the panel charged with updating the *Guideline*, in 1998 Robert Goldenberg and Lorraine Klerman, director and codirector respectively of the Smoke-Free Families National Program Office, organized a conference of experts in the field to define the key elements of effective treatment in the prenatal setting. As a result of the consensus reached at the conference, the 2000 *Guideline* included the first evidence-based recommendation for pregnant smokers, an adaptation of the 5-As that adds five to ten minutes of counseling from a trained prenatal-care provider and distribution of pregnancy-tailored self-help materials.

According to Ralph W. Hale, executive vice president of the American College of Obstetricians and Gynecologists (ACOG), whose members provide most obstetric care in the United States, "These new guidelines provide confirmation that obstetricians and gynecologists need to make tobacco treatment a routine part of prenatal care." ACOG has formally endorsed and disseminated these new guidelines to its members.

Building on this endorsement, Cathy Melvin, who directs the Smoke-Free Families National Dissemination Office, worked with the Smoke-Free Families National Program Office, ACOG's leadership, Robert Wood Johnson Foundation staff members, other funders, and government agencies to form the National Partnership to Help Pregnant Smokers Quit—a group of forty funding, professional, and service organizations that have joined forces to reduce the number of pregnant women who smoke, from an estimated 12–20 percent in 2000 to 2 percent or less by 2010. The Partnership has developed a plan to change practice patterns and health care systems and policies, and to reach pregnant smokers directly through media campaigns.[11] The Partnership was launched in the spring of 2002, and the Foundation is supporting it with a $5 million grant.

—ᴡ— Building Capacity: Managed Care and Systems-Based Approaches

Both the original 1996 tobacco treatment *Guideline* and the 2000 update pointed out that "the success of any tobacco dependence treatment strategy or effort cannot be divorced from the health care system in which it is embedded." The updated *Guideline* recommends creating a culture in which failure to treat tobacco use constitutes an inappropriate standard of health care; it suggests that:

- Every clinic should have a tobacco-user identification system.

- All health care systems should provide education, resources, and feedback to promote provider interventions.

- Clinical sites should dedicate staff members to provide tobacco-dependence treatment and assess the delivery of this treatment in staff performance evaluations.

- Insurers and managed care organizations should reimburse clinicians and specialists for delivering effective tobacco-dependence treatments.

These recommendations emphasized that provider training and knowledge of best practices were necessary (but not complete) ingredients for success.

The Foundation's initial capacity-building efforts centered on its six-year Addressing Tobacco in Managed Care program, launched in 1997 to capitalize on the unique potential and growing reach of managed health care plans. This $7 million national program funds both a National Technical Assistance Office and a program of applied research. The purpose of the National Technical Assistance Office, directed and co-funded by the American Association of Health Plans, is to help institutionalize best-practice tobacco treatments through hands-on technical assistance, an online clearinghouse for practical tools and resource guides, an awards program to recognize tobacco-control leadership, and regular surveys to monitor progress. The research program, codirected by Michael Fiore and Susan Curry, field-tests a variety of promising systems changes under real-world conditions and in varied types of managed care plan.

Both arms of the program have contributed to capacity building. The annual meetings, the awards program, and research grants helped to keep tobacco cessation on managed care's radar screen and quality improvement priority list during turbulent times. Surveys conducted by the American Association of Health Plans in 1997 and 2000 showed increases in the proportion of plans requiring smoking cessation status in patient charts (from 61 to 83 percent); using computerized databases to identify smokers (12 to 27 percent); offering provider tobacco-cessation training (16 to 22 percent); and providing part-time or full-time staff for tobacco control (7 to 23 percent).[12]

The first round of research grants generated new knowledge about the impact of changing the structure of tobacco benefits, provider training and incentives, and other systems.[13] For instance, the Group Health Cooperative (Bob Clement's health plan, with more than six hundred thousand enrollees) launched an initiative to record patient tobacco use status and provider advice to quit as part of an automated billing system. Performance feedback and senior-level incentives were added to foster compliance. Documentation of tobacco use status rose from 7.5 percent of primary care visits to 82 percent; the number of smokers who, like Clement, were advised to quit, rose in a similarly dramatic manner.

Much has been learned as well from the plans singled out for Tobacco Control Achievement Awards. For instance, building on *Guideline* recommendations, HealthPartners, one of three large managed care organizations in the Minneapolis–St. Paul area, evaluated a series of financial incentives and bonus payments on the basis of simple measures and goals. "We made tobacco use a vital sign, and the use of this sign by physicians was a primary goal for financial rewards," says Leif Solberg, HealthPartners's research director and longtime tobacco-cessation investigator.

To receive the bonus, a clinical group must document that its members asked at least 80 percent of its patients about their smoking status and that they provided smoking-cessation advice and assessment (the first and second A's of the 2000 *Guideline*) in 80 percent of the identified smokers. Between 1996 and 1997, the average rate of asking rose from 49 percent to 56 percent, while the rate of quit-smoking advice increased even more substantially. "Although none of the groups earned the bonus the first year, several came very close and most came to us wanting to learn how to put more effective smoking-cessation systems in place," Solberg says. "It was clear that providing the measurement tools and the financial incentives was playing out as we had hoped it would." Two years later, four medical groups received bonuses.

More important, HealthPartners' efforts were having a positive effect on smokers. Nearly 17 percent of the organization's smokers reported having quit during the first sixteen months of the system's installation, compared with only 3.7 percent in the sixteen months before this system started. A follow-up analysis showed that four and a half years after the system was installed, 25 percent of the smokers surveyed had not had a cigarette since their last contact with their primary care clinic, and a third of those who quit had not been smoking for at least a year.[14]

To cut down smoking by pregnant women, Aetna U.S. Healthcare, a 2001 National Tobacco Control Achievement Award recipient, encouraged all of its obstetrical care providers to promote smoking cessation at each patient visit as part of a coordinated, systems-based maternity management program. The program offered pregnant smokers an individualized cessation regimen and provided self-help materials, a video, and a series of follow-up mailings. Forty-five percent of the women who took part quit smoking completely, and 36 percent cut their daily smoking by half or more.

To help ensure that every American prenatal-care provider has similar tools, training, and technical assistance, the Smoke-Free Families National Dissemination Office maintains a Web-based clearinghouse of materials, pregnancy-tailored self-help quitting aids, and links to other organizations offering training. The office is conducting limited studies of systems changes and policy changes and has joined with other members of the National Partnership to Help Pregnant Smokers Quit to provide onsite technical assistance to practitioners and administrators in a variety of health care systems across the country.

—⚒— Boosting Market Demand Among Health Care Purchasers, Policy Makers, and Consumers

Unless there is a demand, or market pull, for tobacco-cessation interventions, neither strengthening the science base nor increasing the capacity of the health care system to deliver effective interventions is going to create the widespread use of smoking-cessation therapy that is needed to reduce the smoking rate substantially. Unless health care purchasers—from companies and governments to individuals—and policy makers reward providers and health plans for making tobacco intervention a priority, physicians and health plans have little incentive to invest in closing the gap that now exists between what we know and what we do. Without clear economic incentives or consumer demand, purchasers and policy makers have found little cause to reimburse or mandate best-practice care for nicotine addiction.

The efforts of The Robert Wood Johnson Foundation to stimulate market demand began with work to make tobacco intervention one of the core measures used by the National Committee on Quality Assurance (NCQA) to grade overall health plan quality for its annual Health Plan Employer Data and Information Set, or HEDIS, report cards. NCQA, a not-for-profit organization often referred to as the watchdog of the managed care industry, developed the HEDIS report card to help health care buyers select the highest-quality health plans.

In 1995, through a Robert Wood Johnson Foundation grant to the Center for the Advancement of Health, more than four hundred tobacco-control researchers and public health and managed care leaders across the country were surveyed about the best empirically based tobacco measures for use in the HEDIS report card. The consensus favored measuring whether health plans routinely asked about and recorded tobacco use. But since this would require costly chart audits, NCQA chose another of the options recommended: asking HMO-enrolled smokers participating in the annual HEDIS survey if they had been advised by any provider to quit in the past year. Tobacco-cessation experts were ecstatic. "This was the first time there was anything having to do with a behavioral risk factor being put into HEDIS, so it was a huge change," says Corinne Husten, epidemiology branch chief in the CDC's Office on Smoking and Health. "The *Guideline* and HEDIS are playing off each other—health plans want to look good on the HEDIS measures, and they can turn to the *Guideline* for help."

Although the HEDIS report card was not as successful as had been hoped in propelling a shift from cost-based to quality-based health care purchasing overall, HEDIS measures were believed to help advance quality improvement efforts in several areas, including tobacco intervention. The tobacco-reporting measure was adopted by HEDIS in 1996, and first reports appeared in 1997. In 1997, in the 375 or so HMOs that report their HEDIS scores, the percentage of smokers who received advice to quit was 61 percent—about 10 percent higher than in the population as a whole. By 2002, the percentage had risen to 65 percent. The Robert Wood Johnson Foundation funded a small study in 1999 exploring how to strengthen the HEDIS tobacco measure by asking patients not just whether they had received advice (the first A in the 5-A approach) but also whether they had received any assistance (the fourth A) in the form of counseling or medication. NCQA formally adopted this new measure—that is, asking smokers whether their health plans offered them tobacco-cessation counseling or medication—in the spring of 2002.

One way to get smokers to quit is to reduce their out-of-pocket costs for insurance copayments, treatment, and pharmaceuticals. The HEDIS tobacco measure, combined with the advocacy of committed managed care leaders, has been credited with reducing copayments for best-practice treatments among smokers enrolled in managed care. There was no reliable national baseline before 1996, but a survey conducted by the American Association of Health Plans in 1997 found that 75 percent of managed care plans were offering full coverage for at least one component of *Guideline*-based counseling or pharmacotherapy—a rate much higher than that reported for indemnity insurers. By 2000, this had risen to 94 percent.[15]

To highlight the need for similar expansion in Medicaid coverage, The Robert Wood Johnson Foundation has funded annual surveys of Medicaid tobacco-dependence treatment coverage since 1998. Although in 1998 all fifty state Medicaid programs covered the costs of treating lung cancer, and forty-six states had sued the tobacco industry to recover these and other tobacco-related Medicaid costs, only twenty-four states then provided any reimbursement for proven tobacco-cessation treatments. Systematically publicizing annual state survey data helped to raise the visibility of these discrepancies and drew attention to the need for expansion of coverage. In 2000, the number of states providing some coverage had risen to thirty-three, although only thirteen provided coverage for the nonmedication counseling services appropriate for most pregnant smokers.[16]

Another way the Foundation sought to stimulate market pull was by clarifying the business case for smoking-cessation programs among public and private health care purchasers, including employers.

Nowhere is the business case stronger than for pregnant smokers: every dollar spent on the 5-A intervention for a pregnant smoker saves about three dollars in reduced neonatal intensive care costs. Cathy Melvin, director of the Smoke-Free Families' Dissemination Office, and Kathleen Adams, an Emory University health economist, were convinced that giving states and health plans a clear picture of their actual costs could make a difference, so they set about making the most of this potential payoff. "No one had ever truly done an estimate of what it costs each year, in direct health care dollars, for pregnant women to smoke," Melvin said. "We wanted to raise awareness of those costs, and to be able to use these estimates to demonstrate the cost-effectiveness of treatment." With funds from The Robert Wood Johnson Foundation, the two researchers developed software (now available through the CDC) that a state, region, or health plan can use to estimate the actual costs of smoking during pregnancy and the potential short-term savings that it could realize.

To help document the business case for employers, the Foundation funded Kenneth Warner, a University of Michigan health economist, to develop a detailed cost-benefit analysis for employers.[17] This study found that a smoking-cessation program returns a third of its costs in the first year through lower health care expenditures and reduced absenteeism and breaks even after about three years—a period shorter than the three-and-a-half-year tenure of the average employee in the United States. Yet a 1997 survey funded by the Foundation and conducted by the Partnership for Prevention, a Washington, D.C.-based organization that works to increase the resources for disease prevention and promotion, found that not even a third of employers offered insurance coverage for smoking cessation.[18] These studies point to the need for new efforts aimed at employers, who select and shape the health benefits for more than 152 million employees and their families. In a follow-up survey co-funded by The Robert Wood Johnson Foundation and the CDC, the Partnership for Prevention is investigating how best to motivate employers to expand their smoking restrictions and treatment benefits.

But of all the activities needed to increase market pull, perhaps the most important and most neglected is translating the smoker's desires to quit into a demand for proven treatment services. Pregnant smokers are a prime example.

Despite the evidence of the effectiveness of a counseling-centered 5-A approach, and the strong interest of prenatal-care providers in offering this help, significant barriers to the demand for treatment exist among the smokers themselves, according to focus groups conducted by the public relations firm Porter Novelli. "Pregnant smokers told us that they knew the risks of smoking to themselves and their babies, but they didn't believe any real help was available to them, especially not from their doctors or nurses." said Ed Maibach, director of social marketing at Porter Novelli. "Most felt that their prenatal-care providers would give them more 'attitude' than empathy or real help to quit. As a result, several didn't even confess to being smokers."

Increasing demand of pregnant smokers will require promotions and campaigns that create an expectation of real and nonjudgmental help, along with parallel efforts to steer providers away from guilt- and fear-arousing tactics toward empathy and effective counseling. A marketing initiative, soon to be launched by Smoke-Free Families and Porter Novelli for the National Partnership to Help Pregnant Smokers Quit, will aim at doing just that.

Pregnant smokers aren't the only ones who do not ask about effective treatment. Many people, it appears, do not realize that smoking-cessation treatment may be covered by insurance. A study conducted jointly by Blue Cross Blue Shield of Minnesota and Minnesota-based HealthPartners under the Addressing Tobacco in Managed Care program found that only a minority of eligible smokers who were offered expanded coverage for Zyban and nicotine replacement actually made use of the benefit. Another Addressing Tobacco in Managed Care study found that providers did not consistently encourage the smokers they saw to take advantage of health plan benefits. Similarly, surveys of patients and providers in two states with very broad Medicaid coverage (nicotine gum, patch, Zyban, and counseling), conducted as part of the year 2001 Medicaid coverage survey, found that the vast majority of patients and providers were unaware of the benefits available.[19] "These findings are disturbing," says Helen Schauffler, who directed the survey. "These states have adopted the most effective policies, but this is all for naught if providers and patients don't even know about them."

—ᴠᴠ— Lessons Learned and Challenges Ahead

Perhaps the most important lesson from the Foundation's work to close the gap between best practice and usual care in tobacco cessation has been that major change is unlikely to come about quickly or from efforts on any single front. Instead, closing the gap takes a combination of improving the scientific basis for and knowledge of effective tobacco-cessation treatments, building the capacity of health care systems to deliver proven best practices, and building a market and a demand for them. There has been encouraging progress on each front, but major change requires sustained, coordinated efforts across the board. As with most social issues, the investments of a single funder pale in comparison to the investment of government and to the need. Most foundations work by leverage. This includes not only strategic partnering but also finding the right points, such as the HEDIS tobacco measure, that can lead to an across-the-board domino effect. Several other, more specific, lessons have emerged as well:

- Scientific evidence alone cannot motivate practice or policy. In the tobacco treatment area, just having a *Guideline* has not been enough. Behind each of the changes linked to the *Guideline* (such as the HEDIS measure or expanded Medicaid and managed care treatment coverage) has been a focused and deliberate effort to translate the science of the *Guideline* into a rationale for practice improvement or policy change.

- The difficulty that many providers have in translating research done in an idealized clinical setting into their own real-world practice has made it clear that we need to work more creatively not only to get research into practice and also to get practice into research, so that interventions are designed *from the beginning* to fit the constraints and capitalize on the unique resources of the actual practice setting.

- Capacity building in a broken health care system is hard, and major systems change—even systems overhaul—is essential if treating tobacco addiction is to become a part of routine health care. This is the same conclusion reached by the 2001 Institute of Medicine report *Crossing the Quality Chasm,* which decried a health care financing and reimbursement system that is "toxic to prevention."[20]

■ The experience of trying to increase the use of tobacco-dependence treatments by the majority of smokers who try to quit has underscored the need to find new ways to build consumer demand and to make a stronger (or clearer) business case for best practices. Judging from recent consumer-driven expansion in coverage for and use of complementary medicine remedies, focusing more on the consumer seems essential. If we are serious about creating more people like Bob Clement, smokers must be actively involved in efforts to improve access to, and use of, proven treatments. Boosting consumer demand requires doing a better job of promoting the treatments that already exist as well as making them more effective and appealing.

■ Finally, the past two decades of research have given us not just the federal clinical practice *Guideline* for helping addicted smokers quit, but also a new set of community guidelines for broader strategies to promote cessation, including raising tobacco prices, strengthening smoking restrictions, launching media campaigns, and reducing smokers' out-of-pocket costs for proven cessation treatments.[21] The Foundation's continuing goal and challenge will be to expand the implementation of both sets of guidelines and to find creative ways to capitalize on the synergy between proven clinical, public health, and policy approaches to prevention and cessation. Only through such a comprehensive approach can we achieve the goals of preventing tobacco-caused death and disease, and improving health and health care for all Americans.

Notes

1. "Bob Clement" is a pseudonym.
2. *Substance Abuse: The Nation's Number One Problem. Key Indicators for Policy.* The Robert Wood Johnson Foundation, 1995.
3. Centers for Disease Control and Prevention. "Cigarette Smoking Among Adults—United States. 1995." *Morbidity and Mortality Weekly Report,* 1997, *46,* 1217–1220.

4. Fiore, M. C., and others (Tobacco Use and Dependence Clinical Practice Guideline Panel, Staff, and Consortium Representatives). "A Clinical Practice Guideline for Treating Tobacco Use and Dependence: A U.S. Public Health Service Report." *Journal of the American Medical Association,* 2000, *283,* 3244–3254.

5. U.S. Public Health Service. "Treating Tobacco Use and Dependence: A Clinical Practice Guideline." (AHRQ publication no. 00–0032) U.S. Department of Health and Human Services, 2000. (www.ahrq.gov)

6. National Cancer Institute. "Population-Based Smoking Cessation." (NIH publication no. 00–4892) U.S. Department of Health and Human Services, 2000.

7. Ferry, L. H., Grission, L. M., and Rinfola, P. S. "Tobacco-Dependence Curricula in U.S. Undergraduate Medical Education." *Journal of the American Medical Association,* 1999, *282,* 825–832.

8. Warner, K., Smith, R., Smith, D., and Fries, B. "Health and Economic Implications of a Worksite Smoking-Cessation Program: A Simulation Analysis." *Journal of Occupational and Environmental Medicine,* 1996, *38,* 981–992; Harris, J. and others, "Expanding Health Insurance Coverage for Smoking Cessation Treatments," *American Journal of Health Promotion,* 2001, *15,* 350–356.

9. *Substance Abuse . . .* (1995).

10. Kottke, T., and others. "Attributes of Successful Smoking Cessation Interventions in Medical Practice: A Meta-Analysis of 39 Controlled Trials." *Journal of the American Medical Association,* 1988, *259,* 2883–2889.

11. "National Partnership to Help Pregnant Smokers Quit: Action Plan." (Unpublished) The Robert Wood Johnson Foundation, 2002.

12. McPhillips-Tangum, C. "Results from the First Annual Survey on Addressing Tobacco in Managed Care." Tobacco Control supplement to vol. 7, S11–13, 1998; McPhillips-Tangum, C. "Addressing Tobacco in Managed Care Survey of Health Plans." Paper presented at the fourth annual Addressing Tobacco in Managed Care conference, Nashville, Tenn., February, 2001.

13. Curry, S. and others. "Addressing Tobacco in Managed Care," *Nicotine and Tobacco Research,* 2002, 4 Supp: S1–S45.

14. Ibid.

15. McPhillips-Tangum (1998 and 2001).

16. Centers for Disease Control. "State Medicaid Coverage for Tobacco-Dependence Treatments—United States, 1998 and 2000. *Morbidity and Mortality Weekly Report,* 2001, *50,* 979–982.

17. Warner, Smith, Smith, and Fries (1996).

18. Partnership for Prevention. "Why Invest in Disease Prevention?" Washington, D.C.: 1999.

19. Mordavsky, J., and others. "Coverage of Tobacco Dependence Treatments for Pregnant Women Under Medicaid and for Children and Parents Under EPSDT." *American Journal of Public Health,* in press.

20. Institute of Medicine. *Crossing the Chasm: A New Health System for the 21st Century.* Washington, D.C.: National Academy Press, 2001.

21. Centers for Disease Control. "The Guide to Community Preventive Services: Tobacco Use and Prevention. Reviews, Recommendations, and Expert Commentary." *American Journal of Preventive Medicine,* supplement to vol. 20, 2002.

7

Combating Alcohol Abuse in Northwestern New Mexico

Gallup's Fighting Back and Healthy Nations Programs

Paul Brodeur

Editors' Introduction

Last year, *The Robert Wood Johnson Foundation Anthology* included a chapter that examined a single Foundation-funded program in Albuquerque, New Mexico, called Recovery High.[1] In this year's *Anthology,* Paul Brodeur, an award-winning author and former staff writer for the *New Yorker,* focuses on one city trying to address what seemed like an intractable problem. In the 1970s and 1980s, Gallup, New Mexico, in the rural northwestern corner of the state, had a frighteningly high rate of alcohol abuse, mostly because of heavy drinking among Native Americans coming to town from the surrounding reservations.

With leadership from a small number of citizens, and building on an eye-opening tragedy, the town slowly but surely became engaged in reducing the high rate of drinking. In the early stage of Gallup's efforts to attack its alcohol problem, the Foundation announced a new program, Fighting Back® It funded local coalitions to develop strategies to reduce substance abuse and to implement communitywide campaigns to address the prob-lem.[2] Local leaders put together a proposal that eventually was funded as one of the fourteen sites of the Fighting Back initiative, even though the Gallup approach was quite distinct from that used in the other thirteen sites. When funding from Fighting Back ended, Gallup's efforts were picked up by the Foundation's Healthy Nations® program, one of two national programs that have supported locally developed strategies to address alcohol abuse problems among Native Americans.[3]

The story of Gallup is a good example of how timely funding from a foundation can help move an agenda of pressing concern to a commu-nity. In fact, The Robert Wood Johnson Foundation's support fit so seam-lessly into the activities under way in Gallup that it is difficult to isolate its role and contribution. The story also shows how much endurance it takes for a local community to address deep-seated, long-term social prob-lems. Foundation resources can be helpful, but strong leadership and local will are essential prerequisites to bring about change.

1. Diehl, D. "Recovery High School." In *To Improve Health and Health Care, Vol. V: The Robert Wood Johnson Foundation Anthology.* San Francisco: Jossey-Bass, 2001.

2. Robert Hughes traces the history of the Foundation's involvement in reducing the harm coming from substance abuse in "Adopting the Substance Abuse Goal: A Story of Philanthropic Decision Making." In *To Improve Health and Health Care 1998-1999: The Robert Wood Johnson Foundation Anthology.* San Francisco: Jossey-Bass, 1999. See also the report on the Fighting Back initiative on The Robert Wood Johnson Foundation's Website (www.rwjf.org).

3. These programs are examined in Brodeur, P. "Programs to Improve the Health of Native Americans." In *To Improve Health and Health Care, Vol. V: The Robert Wood Johnson Foundation Anthology.* San Francisco: Jossey-Bass, 2001.

—℁—Police officers and ambulance drivers called them "popsicles": the people they would find frozen to death as a result of alcoholic stupor on the streets of Gallup, New Mexico, a city of twenty-one thousand inhabitants situated in the seven-thousand-foot-high desert of northwestern New Mexico, where winter temperatures often drop below zero. For years, Gallup billed itself as "the Indian Capital of the World," because it served as the principal shopping center for thousands of Native Americans, who drove into the city from surrounding reservations on weekends. During the 1970s and 1980s, however, Gallup also became known as "Drunk Town, USA," as statistics suggested that alcohol abuse there had reached epidemic proportions. By 1988, more than thirty-four thousand people were being picked up each year in Gallup for public intoxication and detained for up to twelve hours in the city's crammed and squalid "drunk tank," under a New Mexico protective custody program that was begun, in 1973, after public drunkenness was decriminalized. By comparison, just over a thousand people were held in protective custody for drunkenness that same year in Albuquerque, 130 miles to the east, which has nearly twenty times the population.[1]

Very few of those being picked up in Gallup were residents of the city. More than 90 percent of them were Native Americans—mostly Navajos from the vast twenty-five-thousand-square-mile Navajo Nation reservation of some 175,000 inhabitants, which lies to the north and east of Gallup, in McKinley and San Juan Counties, and to the north and west of the city, in Arizona.[2] The detainees also included residents of the Zuni pueblo, the Acoma pueblo, and the Laguna pueblo, all independent nations with sizeable Indian populations. A federal law prohibiting the sale of liquor to Indians had been repealed by Congress in 1953, but the Navajo, Zuni, Acoma, and Laguna continued to ban liquor on their reservations.

As a result, Native Americans from the surrounding area came to Gallup to drink, and the liquor industry in Gallup—a city prone to boom-and-bust cycles because of the rise and fall in the demand for the coal and uranium that had long been mined in the region—seized the opportunity to take advantage of Gallup's unique situation as a "wet" border town. During the next three and a half decades,

Gallup's economy was largely based not only upon selling groceries, goods, and services to Native Americans but also upon creating an environment that encouraged them to drink.

By 1987, sixty-one establishments in Gallup had been issued liquor licenses, which was more than five times the number allotted under a New Mexico law permitting only one license for every two thousand inhabitants. Among them were twenty-five drive-up windows where one could buy liquor without leaving one's car.[3] Bars in the city were open seven days a week, from 7:00 A.M. until 2:00 A.M. Wine fortified with brandy to make it 19 percent alcohol came into Gallup from California twice a month in tanker trucks that each carried fifty-five hundred gallons.[4] Many of the city's most prominent citizens not only owned bars, restaurants, and liquor distribution outlets but also had been elected to public office and appointed to various municipal and civic organizations. One of these families had been bottling and selling a fortified wine called Garden DeLuxe (known as "Garden Death" on the street) since 1946. By 1987, the liquor industry had become one of Gallup's economic mainstays, reporting $14.2 million in sales—more taxable earnings than in the finance, insurance, and real estate industries combined.[5]

In addition to permitting easy access to liquor, Gallup had become a civic enabler for alcohol abusers in other ways. The city had twenty-one pawnshops (compared with twenty-four in all of Albuquerque), a blood plasma donation center, and two bottle recycling centers, which gave problem drinkers a way to pick up quick and easy cash. Gallup also had three church-operated soup kitchens and two free overnight shelters, compared with five soup kitchens and seven shelters in Albuquerque.[6] Together with a revolving-door protective custody program, which amounted to a free overnight stay in the Gallup jail, these facilities offered little incentive for alcoholics picked up in Gallup to seek treatment for their disease.

What resulted from all this can be ascertained from the mortality data collected by the National Institute on Alcohol Abuse and Alcoholism (NIAAA), for McKinley County—site of the largest portion of the Navajo reservation in New Mexico—of which Gallup is the county seat. As early as the mid-1970s, McKinley

County was ranked by the NIAAA as the worst of all 3,106 counties in the United States for alcohol-related mortality.[7] In 1974, the mortality rate from cirrhosis in McKinley County was 2.3 times as high as the national average, the alcohol-induced mortality rate was 9.8 times as high, and the mortality rate from all alcohol-related causes was 3.7 times as high. For the three-year period 1974–76, the mortality rates of McKinley County residents for selected substance abuse-related causes were between 184 percent and 337 percent higher than those for New Mexico residents as a whole.[8]

According to the NIAAA, McKinley County ranked first in the list of per capita deaths from chronic alcoholism, at nineteen times the nationwide rate. Alcohol-related homicides and suicides were three times the national rate. During the 1970s and 1980s, the county's drunken-driving death rate was seven times the U.S. rate.[9] One out of every twenty licensed drivers in McKinley County had received at least two drunken-driving citations since 1984.[10] From 1982 through 1987, McKinley had the highest rate of alcohol-related traffic fatalities among New Mexico's thirty-three counties.[11] During the three-year period between 1986 and 1988, the county led the nation in motor vehicle deaths.[12] Between 1983 and 1988, some 660 Navajos died on highways in northwestern New Mexico.[13]

The U.S. Public Health Service's Indian Health Service estimated that there were fifty-five thousand problem drinkers on the Navajo reservation.[14] A survey of Navajo seventh and eighth graders found that 58 percent of them had one or more parents who were alcoholics.[15] Sporadic binge drinking and chronic drinking were strongly associated with child neglect and abuse, and with domestic violence on the reservation. Fetal Alcohol Syndrome (FAS) had been found to be the leading major birth defect in the region, particularly among Navajos, in whom FAS children were born to an average of six per thousand women of child-bearing age.[16] Alcohol had begun to appear at many of the Navajo traditional ceremonies. "We are hanging on to our traditions by a string," one community worker said, "and alcohol can break that string." In May 1988, Mother Teresa added Gallup to her itinerary of forsaken places.[17]

Such was the background for a stark assessment contained in a report issued by officials of the Marin Institute for the Prevention of Alcohol and Other

Drug Problems, in San Rafael, California. Following a visit to Gallup in 1989, they wrote:

> In all our years of providing consultation and technical assistance to cities dealing with alcohol and drug-related problems, we have never encountered a situation as serious as that facing Gallup, the Native American reservations, and the surrounding region. It is no exaggeration to say that alcohol-related problems are undermining the cultural integrity of the Native American community, and although it could be a difficult concept to accept, in our opinion the situation may be described as observable genocide. We concur with the *Albuquerque Tribune*'s assessment that Gallup is "a town under the influence." Never before have we observed such a high concentration of liquor establishments in such a small area. Never before have we seen a town's power structure dominated by liquor dealers and their associates. Never before have we seen wine fortified with brandy brought into a town by the tanker truckload.[18]

—w— The Beginning of a Turnaround

In 1986, a fifty-eight-year-old Hispanic named Edward Muñoz was elected as mayor of Gallup on a platform that called for taking drastic action to resolve the city's alcohol-abuse crisis. Muñoz, who has close-cropped silver hair that fits his head like a helmet, had previously served as mayor from 1958 to 1969 and subsequently gone into the auto-wrecking business. His own father had been run over and killed by a drunk driver in Gallup in 1947, but like many of his fellow citizens he was conditioned to accept the ravages of alcoholism as something he and other residents of the city simply had to live with. "People had become so accustomed to alcohol abuse in Gallup that they stopped seeing it," he said not long ago. "I didn't understand the extent of the problem myself until I went into the auto-wrecking business. Then, when I saw the hideous accidents caused by drunken driving, I realized that something had to be done."

Small in stature but formidably feisty, Muñoz ran a no-holds-barred campaign. He put out a flyer that called for legislation to impose a stiff tax on the sale of liquor, close down drive-up windows, and stop liquor sales on Sunday. He charged that the city's drunk tank was "inhumane" and attacked Gallup's liquor merchants—some of whom were old friends and former mayors—for helping to perpetuate the cycle of alcohol abuse. "We say that an alcoholic has a disease, but we bottle, sell, and tax this disease," he wrote in one of his campaign pamphlets. In an election against four other candidates, he won with 30 percent of the vote.

Once in office, Muñoz sought help from the Northwest New Mexico Council of Governments, an association of ten local governments in the three adjoining counties of McKinley (where Gallup is located), San Juan, and Cibola; they form the northwest quadrant of the state and an area larger than Massachusetts, Rhode Island, and Connecticut combined. Funded by grants and money contributed by member city, county, state, and tribal governments, the council was created to afford a means for the member governments to work together in areas of shared concern. Council staff members began collecting data on Gallup's alcohol-abuse crisis, as well as on the corollary cost to various government agencies—among them police departments, ambulance services, and hospitals—that had to respond to and deal with the crisis.

They also consulted Philip May, an expert in the field of Indian alcoholism, who is a professor of sociology and psychiatry and director of the Center on Alcoholism, Substance Abuse, and Addiction at the University of New Mexico, in Albuquerque. May made research available showing that Indians drinking in a border town near a reservation on which the sale and consumption of liquor were banned followed a pattern of binge drinking similar to that of college students. His studies also indicated that much of the drinking in Gallup was anxiety-driven on the part of Native Americans seeking escape from a depressed and socially marginal existence that resulted largely from a poverty level of 40 percent on the Navajo reservation, and an unemployment rate that ranged from 30 to 75 percent. In addition, May shattered the prevalent myth that American Indians had a biological weakness for the effects of alcohol. "This myth has no basis in fact," he told the council staff members, explaining that scientific studies had found Indians to metabolize alcohol at the same rate as non-Indians.[19]

In 1987, at the urging of Mayor Muñoz, the Northwest New Mexico Council of Governments conducted a survey to determine whether residents of McKinley County would be willing to accept a tax on liquor to be spent on alcohol prevention and treatment programs. The response was overwhelming, with

80 percent of the people polled supporting a 5 percent increase, which would bring the total excise tax on liquor to 15 percent.

At about the same time, Dr. David Conejo, chief executive of the Rehoboth McKinley Christian Hospital, a private hospital in Gallup that operated the city's only in-patient alcohol treatment program, became concerned about the program's long waiting list and decided that the time had arrived for the hospital to become more deeply involved. In the summer of 1988, he invited a group of health care professionals and concerned citizens to discuss Gallup's alcohol problem. At the meeting, Dr. Thomas Carmany, the hospital's chief of pathology, who had become weary of performing autopsies on alcoholic victims of cirrhosis, reminded the group that the hospital's mission was to provide a health care system that was "responsive to all people." He then issued a blunt challenge: "How long are you willing to keep stepping over bodies?"

Mayor Muñoz and the group convened by Conejo began meeting with tribal leaders, city and county officials, school board members, health providers, parents, and others who had become interested in the anti-liquor movement. They also met with state lawmakers, who, for the most part, repeated time-worn excuses to the effect that the alcohol problem in Gallup was too big and too far gone to solve, and that Gallup had always been and would continue to be a wide-open drinking town. One of the most powerful men in New Mexico politics, Raymond Sanchez, who was the Democratic Speaker of the House, minced no words. "You're not going to change things in Gallup," he told staff members of the Council of Governments. "And the legislature has no money for you."[20]

In September 1987, Gallup's indefatigable Mayor Muñoz called for an "Alcohol Awareness Week," spending his own money to print a thousand T-shirts for an anti-alcohol fun run. Highlight of the week was a Saturday parade with thirty-six entries from various civic, religious, and school groups. A float representing the Rehoboth McKinley Christian Hospital showed mannequins spurting fake blood from a wrecked car. The Gallup Christian Center float featured a shack inhabited by a drunk who refused to allow his family inside. The Grim Reaper glared from another display. Still another float showed a cemetery filled with crying children. No member of the Gallup City Council showed up to watch the parade.

Undiscouraged, Muñoz renewed his assault upon Gallup's liquor industry and its captains. "It may be a legal business, but it's immoral," he told the *Albuquerque Tribune,* which ran a scathing six-part series called "Gallup: The Town Drunk," in the early autumn of 1988. "How can these guys say they are not responsible? People don't get run over by trains, hit by cars, and freeze to death by drinking milk."[21] Later in the series, Muñoz expanded his criticism to include the entire city. After pointing out that many people felt the economy of Gallup would fail if large amounts of liquor were not sold and consumed in the city, he declared, "If this is the case, we have a sick community."[22]

The *Tribune*'s six-part series was graphic, to say the least, with color photographs showing bystanders standing over the body of a man who had staggered out of a bar and into a hit-and-run accident; the freshly snow-dusted body of a drunken man, frozen to death at dawn, a few yards from a police station; and a dead sixteen-year-old Navajo girl, killed in a drunken-driving one-car rollover, with her hand still clutching a beer can. (Not surprisingly, the articles received nationwide attention, with segments on the alcohol crisis in Gallup subsequently being aired on NBC's "Today," ABC's "20/20," and PBS's "On Assignment.") At the time, however, many Gallup citizens responded with outrage, characterizing the accounts as unduly sensational and demanding that *Tribune* editors, reporters, and photographers listen to their complaints. Two hundred of them attended a town hall meeting to vent their wrath. After listening for more than an hour to diatribes critical of the newspaper, Muñoz got to his feet and accused them of being in denial, like many alcoholics, and challenging them to take action to improve the situation in Gallup instead of attacking those who had brought it to public attention.

Impressed by their mayor's courage, some residents of Gallup began to offer Muñoz help with his crusade. Others were distrustful of his motives and resentful of what they considered to be his displays of civic disloyalty. The extent to which the city remained divided would become apparent a year and a half later, when the controversial mayor had to withstand a recall election after he incensed many voters by telling state legislators that unless they passed bills to control drunken driving in New Mexico, he would erect billboards proclaiming the state to be the drunk-driving capital of the world.[23]

Meanwhile, *Tribune* reporters interviewed every lawmaker heading to Santa Fe for the mid-January 1989 opening of the New Mexico legislative session, asking what he or she thought the state could do to help Gallup resolve its alcohol crisis. The answers were discouraging. Most of the lawmakers pointed out that the budget was tight, and that the governor, Garrey Carruthers, had come out against raising taxes for any new programs or facilities. On January 10, the *Tribune* ran an article under a headline that read "No Hope Seen for Anti-Liquor Bills."[24]

That was just four days before a highway accident that forever changed the attitude toward alcohol abuse of the lawmakers in Santa Fe and the residents of Gallup and northwestern New Mexico.

—ⱳ— The Journey for Jovita

Late in the afternoon of January 14, a thirty-two-year-old rodeo rider named Robert Christie, who had been drinking all day, left a Gallup bar with a bottle of vodka in his hand, climbed into his pickup truck, and headed south on a two-lane road toward the Zuni reservation. A short time later, he crashed head-on into a van carrying Kathleen Vega; her sister, Shirley Harry; her twelve-year-old niece, Cheryl; and her infant daughter, Katherine ("Jovita"), who were on their way to a revival meeting. Three-month-old Jovita, who was half Hispanic and half Navajo, was killed instantly, as were Shirley and Cheryl Harry. Christie, whose blood-alcohol level turned out to be more than three times the legal limit, also died at the scene. Only Jovita's mother, Kathleen Vega, survived.[25]

Outrage over the senselessness of the latest highway carnage spread through Gallup, McKinley County, and the Navajo and Zuni reservations. David Conejo, of the Rehoboth McKinley Christian Hospital, reacted by suggesting a citizen's march to Santa Fe, two hundred miles away, in an effort to force New Mexico's legislators to take action. The idea caught on quickly. Earl Tulley, a young and dedicated social and environmental activist, who spoke Navajo, visited chapter houses (community centers) across the reservation, urging his fellow Navajos to participate in the march. Mayor Muñoz and David Conejo's wife, Judith, arranged for the walkers to be housed and fed in churches, chapter houses, tribal buildings, and other shelters along the route of the procession, which was named

"March of Hope: Journey for Jovita." The plan was to walk twenty miles a day for ten days with a group of support vehicles that would enable Navajo senior citizens, called elders, to participate by walking a little of the distance each day and then riding the rest of the way in vans.

Starting on February 10, approximately one hundred people started out on foot, east on Interstate Highway 40, toward Albuquerque. Among them were Hispanics, Navajos, Zunis, and other Native Americans, as well as many white residents of Gallup, including teachers, bankers, and bureaucrats. Their numbers swelled along the way. The new arrivals on the second day included three elderly Navajo women, respectfully called "grandmothers," who had walked twenty-five miles from Mariano Lake to join the march at Thoreau. "They were wearing floppy rubber boots and carrying flimsy little blankets," Muñoz recalled recently. "So we bought them walking shoes and sleeping bags when we got to Grants." Dr. Herbert Mosher, vice president for development at Rehoboth McKinley Christian Hospital, remembered that it started snowing, and that he went up to one of the grandmothers with the idea of dissuading her from continuing in the march. "She made as if she were going to hit me with her walking stick," he recalled. "She was absolutely furious. It turned out that her husband had frozen to death while drunk, and that the husband of one of the other grandmothers had been in a car-train wreck after drinking. Between the three of them, they had lost twelve relatives to alcohol-related disease and accidents."

By the time the marchers reached Santa Fe, on February 20, their number had grown to more than two thousand. Hundreds of other supporters, arriving by car and van, together with dozens of reporters and photographers, were waiting for them on the Capitol steps. Said Muñoz:

> It was the largest demonstration of its kind in New Mexico history, and it caught the politicians in Santa Fe by surprise. The head of the Department of Highways advised Governor Carruthers, who was attending a national governors conference in Kansas City, to return to the capital as quickly as possible, and the legislators called a joint session of the House and Senate to listen to the grievances and demands of the demonstrators. Kathleen Vega spoke first and then embraced Robert Christie's former wife, Marcie, who told the legislators that she had loved her husband but hated his disease. There wasn't a dry eye in the place.

Before the 1989 legislative session was over, the Journey for Jovita had achieved significant success. New Mexico lawmakers earmarked $300,000 from the over-all state appropriations bill to design a regional detoxification and rehabilitation clinic, initially called the Gallup Alcohol Crisis Center, which would replace Gallup's infamous drunk tank. They also enacted a law prohibiting open containers of alcoholic beverage in a motor vehicle. An excise tax bill granting McKinley County the power to hold a local referendum on raising the liquor tax passed the House by a vote of 58–0, and the Senate by 24–0 (the next year, voters in McKinley County approved a 5 percent increase in the excise tax on liquor, whose proceeds would be used to finance construction of the Alcohol Crisis Center). A bill banning drive-up windows at retail liquor outlets in McKinley County and neighboring San Juan County passed the House 57–2 and the Senate 32–2. As the result of a legal technicality, San Juan County was able to avoid having to comply with the law, while the McKinley County Retail Liquor Dealers Association sued to overturn it, on the ground of unfair restraint of trade. The lawsuit failed, however, and the ban against the drive-up windows went into effect in 1992, after residents of the county voted overwhelmingly in favor of it.[26]

—ⵡ— The Robert Wood Johnson Foundation's Fighting Back® Program

The March of Hope: Journey for Jovita galvanized continuing support for alcohol reform in McKinley, San Juan, and Cibola counties. Early in 1990, the Northwest New Mexico Council of Governments received a $200,000 grant from The Robert Wood Johnson Foundation to develop a plan that would enable the three counties to participate in a Foundation program called Fighting Back: Community Initiatives to Reduce Demand for Illegal Drugs and Alcohol. Only fourteen out of more than three hundred community applicants across the nation were selected by the Foundation to receive such planning grants, and the tricounty region was the only one in a rural area.

At the end of August, two hundred citizens, health professionals, public officials, and alcohol-reform activists attended a three-day Regional Substance Abuse Summit Conference in Gallup, where they formulated key elements of a comprehensive plan to attack alcohol abuse in northwestern New Mexico. Many of the ideas and suggestions developed at the conference were integrated into an implementation plan for the second phase of the Fighting Back program, which was being developed by a regional task force (later reduced to a twenty-member core committee), and by the members of half a dozen subcommittees. Initial objectives of the ambitious twenty-component plan included reducing by 25 percent the number of cases of alcohol and drug-related domestic violence, the number of individuals picked up for protective custody because of public intoxication, the number of alcohol and drug-related vehicle accidents and traffic fatalities, and the number of deaths directly or indirectly related to alcohol or drug abuse. The plan also called for reducing the incidence of Fetal Alcohol Syndrome in the region from 3.4 per thousand to 2.0 per thousand.[27]

In 1991, Congress appropriated $1.2 million for three specific projects in northwestern New Mexico. Of this, $900,000 was earmarked for startup operations at the Gallup Alcohol Crisis Center, $200,000 to finance a treatment program in Gallup at the Rehoboth McKinley Christian Hospital's Behavioral Health Services campus, and $100,000 to renovate a Navajo Nation treatment center in the town of Crownpoint, which is a fifty-mile drive northeast of Gallup. Groundbreaking for the Gallup Alcohol Crisis Center took place on August 7. Meanwhile, members of various Fighting Back committees struggled with the difficult task of creating a coordinated regional program for the vast tricounty area. Some idea of the difficulty was described in a paragraph of the Implementation Proposal that the Council of Governments sent to The Robert Wood Johnson Foundation on September 9:

> In northwest New Mexico, the unique challenge is to accomplish this purpose by finding points of order, commonality, and unity within a tremendously diverse regional community, composed of three counties, six municipalities, four Native American nations, a substantial Hispanic population, and seventy-eight small rural communities. These peoples, 180,000 strong, are spread across 15,000 square miles of New Mexico highlands. Any strategy in this region which attempts to unify services and activities around the reduction of substance abuse must deal with multiple jurisdictions and governments, multiple cultures and world views, the unique problems associated with "wet-versus-dry" alcohol availability issues, and

difficult (and often "co-dependent") relationships within and between institutions and communities.[28]

Some of the most important contributions to the Fighting Back Implementation Plan were made by members of a Native American Issues Subcommittee, who believed strongly that alcohol abuse was a community problem, not simply a problem of individual addiction or disease. "The need for a community conscience which admits it has a problem with alcohol abuse is akin to the individual alcoholic overcoming the state of denial and having to admit to himself and others he has a problem with alcohol and that he cannot solve his problem alone," they wrote in a position paper dated July 15, 1991.[29] They also recommended that Fighting Back funds be used to deal with underlying problems, such as intercultural alienation, the disempowerment felt at all levels of the Native American community, and the inadequate and often inappropriate responses of public and private institutions to the needs of Native American people.

Realizing the need for balance between a regional approach and support and empowerment of grassroots communities and organizations, the planners of the Fighting Back program decided to focus their efforts on encouraging creation of community coalitions, called Fighting Back Associations, in ten existing jurisdictional areas with common ethnic, economic, and social ties. In addition to the three counties that made up the overall region, the designated areas were the Zuni, Laguna, and Acoma pueblos, and Indian agencies on the Ramah-Navajo and Eastern Navajo reservations, and in the towns of Shiprock and Fort Defiance. (The Fighting Back Association in Fort Defiance was later transferred to the Indian agency in Chuska.) The initiative called for coordinators trained in all aspects of substance abuse, and working out of field offices, to assist the local Fighting Back Associations in developing individual action plans to address critical needs, such as public awareness; community organizing; relapse prevention; aftercare support systems; prevention of Fetal Alcohol Syndrome and Fetal Alcohol Effect; driving while intoxicated, or DWI; prevention; family counseling; youth development; and environmental risk reduction.

In February 1992, The Robert Wood Johnson Foundation awarded the Northwest New Mexico Council of Governments a $3 million, five-year Fighting Back grant to carry out programs designed to create long-term solutions to the problem of alcohol abuse in the three-county region. Later that year, the core committee reorganized itself into a board of directors known as the Regional Council, whose membership was based upon proportionate representation from each of the subregional Fighting Back Associations. Intent upon maintaining Native American sovereignty, the members of the Regional Council voted to make the Fighting Back program an independent entity. This led to the formation of a non-profit corporation called Northwest New Mexico Fighting Back and, in May 1993, to transfer of The Robert Wood Johnson Foundation grant from the Council of Governments to the newly formed corporation.

Over the next five years, practical considerations dictated that the twenty component projects of the Fighting Back program be scaled back to three: community organizing and mobilization to create and implement local solutions to alcohol abuse, public awareness to educate people in the community about the devastating impact of alcohol abuse, and training community members to facilitate community forums and meetings to discuss issues of concern. Within this framework, Fighting Back volunteers increased education about Fetal Alcohol Syndrome and Fetal Alcohol Effect in the tricounty region; participated in developing a regional computer-based case management system to coordinate referral and tracking of clients; worked with communities to effect a significant decline in alcohol-related traffic accidents; organized a "Sacred Journey to Save Lives March" along Route 44; provided wellness gatherings throughout the region; and developed the Zuni Mountain Realization of Personal Excellence and Strength, or ROPES, course, in Cibola County.

In addition, they established Boys and Girls Clubs in the Navajo town of Tohatchi, thirty miles north of Gallup, and in the Laguna pueblo, which is a hundred miles to the southeast; supported development of youth training in wilderness skills; helped establish the Gallup Youth Center and the Future Family Foundation Center; organized a National Football League Players Association/Navajo Nation Football Camp; staged a statewide Multicultural Red Ribbon Relay Run to bring attention to alcohol and drug abuse; and introduced a spiritually based healing curriculum, called Gathering of Native Americans, or GONA, into several communities. (Participants in GONA examine historical trauma and its relation to alcohol abuse, identify strategies to deal with the problem, and learn how community healing is essential for prevention of alcohol and substance abuse.)

In the realm of policy, the Fighting Back program educated the citizens of Gallup about a referendum that resulted in banning Sunday liquor sales in the city and supported a measure lowering the breath-alcohol count under which someone could be charged with DWI. In addition, the Fighting Back program backed measures mandating jail time for multiple DWI offenders, training for alcohol servers about responsible drinking, and a five-year waiting period for licensing new alcohol outlets.

In 1994, Northwest New Mexico Fighting Back and The Robert Wood Johnson Foundation's Fighting Back National Program Office commissioned Bernard Ellis & Associates, a consulting firm based in Santa Fe, Tennessee, to conduct a review of the extent of substance abuse in McKinley County. According to the report, McKinley County—once the worst county in the United States for alcohol-related mortality—had significantly reduced its alcohol-related death rate from accidents, motor vehicle crashes, homicide, suicide, and cirrhosis.[30] Three years later, a second report by the same consulting firm showed that between 1993 and 1995 cirrhosis mortality in the county was 43 percent lower than between 1974 and 1976. In addition, the report showed that from 1982 to 1995 the alcohol-related fatality or injury crash rate for McKinley County had not only declined significantly but also exceeded the declines in New Mexico over the same period of time.[31]

—ᴡ— The Na'nizhoozhi Center

Na'nizhoozhi, which means "bridge" in Navajo, is the name Navajos gave Gallup because they had to cross bridges over the Rio Puerco to come into town from their reservation. It is also the name that was given to the Gallup Alcohol Crisis Center soon after it opened in September 1992, because the 150-bed protective custody and predetoxification facility is considered to be a bridge to recovery for those who suffer from alcoholism. For that reason, a tile mural of a bridge and the words "Courage to Change, Wisdom to Accept" hang over the entrance of the Center, which has been constructed of red sandstone blocks that match the color of the sandstone bluffs running along the valley corridor in which Gallup is situated.

A collaborative effort to address the alcohol crisis in Gallup and north-western New Mexico, the Na'nizhoozhi Center, Inc., or NCI, was developed by the Navajo and Zuni Nations, the City of Gallup, and McKinley County, with support from the New Mexico state government and the Rehoboth McKinley Christian Hospital. Its construction was financed by a $1.6 million bond issued by the City of Gallup, which has since been retired by proceeds from the increased excise tax on liquor, and its annual operational cost of approximately $1 million is covered by the federal government and transferred to the Navajo Nation through the government's Indian Health Service. Intoxicated adults who have been taken into protective custody by police or other law enforcement officials are held at the center for at least twenty-four hours before being released into the custody of a sober relative or friend. Local hospitals, families, and citizens can also bring intoxicated people to NCI, which can offer protective custody for one hundred men and twenty-five women who are age eighteen or older. A court order, or three protective custody admissions in a thirty-day period, result in a five-day emergency commitment, as required by New Mexico statutes for detoxification. Physicians can also request the five-day hold, during which patients receive counseling and attend meetings based upon the Alcoholics Anonymous model. Patients can remain longer if they volunteer to participate in the Center's short-term adult shelter program, or in its twenty-three-day traditional healing program.

The traditional healing program—the first ever for a government-funded detoxification center—is known as the Hi'ina'ah Bits'os (Eagle Plume) Society. (The name refers to the story of twin Navajo warriors who visited their father, the Sun, looking for self-identify and knowledge, and who were given a sacred Eagle Plume for protection by Spider Woman.) The goal of the program, which is directed by Navajo medicine men, is to promote healthy behavior through the clanship system (K'e)—a method of identification that ties Navajo families to specific locations on the vast reservation, and to the Beauty Way philosophy, which entails a lifelong journey of healing, empowerment, and resilience. How to live a positive life is revealed through ancient Navajo myths and by participating in traditional ceremonies that employ drumming, chanting, praying, and use of corn pollen pouches. A Navajo basket teachings project seeks to collect and share legends that help prevent and treat alcohol abuse. As part of the traditional healing program, the Na'nizhoozhi Center provides hogans for men and women, sweat lodges, and a cooking area for preparing traditional Navajo food, such as roast mutton and fry bread. In keeping with the clanship system, the Center's clients and the its 125-member staff, the great majority of whom are Navajo, think of themselves as family members and refer to each other as "relatives."

It was Raymond Daw who came up with the idea of calling clients at the Na'nizhoozhi Center relatives. Daw, a forty-nine-year-old Navajo from Houck, Arizona, has nearly fifteen years of experience in dealing with alcohol and substance abuse in the Navajo Nation. Between 1988 and 1991, he was clinical director of the Navajo Department of Behavioral Health Services, where he was in charge of treatment programs. Between 1992 and 1993, he was assistant director of operations for the Na'nizhoozhi Center, and since 1994 he has been executive director. (From 1996 to 1999, he was executive director of Northwest New Mexico Fighting Back.) A soft-spoken man who wears his long hair tied in a traditional Navajo bun, he has a master's degree in counseling and psychology from the University of New Mexico, and some interesting ideas about how to treat alcohol abuse among his Navajo relatives:

> When I was clinical director of the Navajo Department of Behavioral Health Services, I saw my field counselors working from the standard Alcoholics Anonymous model, and realized that the AA method was not successful in treating Navajos because it was not culturally sensitive to their ways. Once I became director here at NCI, I saw a need to institute a traditional healing program. For this reason, I encouraged two young medicine men to proceed with the development of the Eagle Plume Society, which I believe has played a large role in the success we have had in reducing the rate of protective custody admissions. As far as I'm concerned, one of the biggest problems we face in the future will be pressure upon us to place too much emphasis on science-based treatment—for example, chemical and drug intervention. Such interventions have been designed for dense urban populations with ready access to monitoring facilities, but not for the kind of rural population that lives in the open spaces of the huge Navajo reservation. In addition, they are not culturally appropriate for the Navajo people.

Daw's high regard for traditional healing is echoed by Matthew Kelley, a tall, graying, and intensely enthusiastic man who has been clinical director in charge of treatment programs at the Na'nizhoozhi Center since 1994. Kelley's early background is eclectic, to say the least. After graduating from the University of Alaska in 1974, he became a smoke jumper during the summers and studied transcendental meditation at a Swiss monastery for seven winters. He then studied biofeedback at the Menninger Clinic, in Topeka, Kansas, and received a degree in clinical psychiatry from the Saybrook Institute, in San Francisco. Later, he worked at the Navajo Nation headquarters, in Window Rock, conducting a study on neurotherapy feedback for problem drinkers.

"A problem drinker drinks because he doesn't feel good about himself when he's sober," Kelley said not long ago, as he sat at his desk in a small office whose walls are covered with drawings—some of them remarkably accomplished—that have been done by patients at the Center. He continues:

> The important thing is to get him to feel better about himself against the odds. The AA model, which is based upon guilt and disclosure, doesn't work with Navajos, who are among the most spiritually inclined of all the Native American peoples. What is needed is the inner and cultural empowerment afforded by the kind of traditional healing program we encourage here. It can change the low brainwave frequencies and racing brainwave patterns that are common among alcoholics. A Navajo patient coming out of a sweat lodge exhibits such changes. He feels better in mind and body—reborn, if you will. So there's a new paradigm in the making here at NCI. We're in the process of transforming this place from a detox center into a place of healing.

There is little doubt that the Na'nizhoozhi Center has played a significant role in reducing the number of protective custody admissions that were occurring annually in Gallup. During its first year of operation, admissions were 26 percent lower than admissions to the drunk tank in previous years, and by 1998 the number was about half the annual levels that had occurred during the 1980s. By that time, there was also a 33 percent drop in emergency room visits for alcohol-related causes at the Gallup Indian Medical Center, and more than a 60 percent decrease in the number of winter exposure deaths resulting from alcohol abuse. The Center has also been able to give a clearer picture of the chronic alcoholic population in the region, including the average blood alcohol level of public intoxicants, and their chapter residence on the Navajo reservation—a piece of information vital in making treatment referrals and follow-up visits.

A further example of the value of the Na'nizhoozhi Center as a data collector and early warning system can be found in the results of a 1999 study it conducted on the ingestion of Ocean, a combination of hairspray and water popular among many substance abusers in northwestern New Mexico. (Typical hair spray contains 70 percent or more specially denatured alcohol not intended for human consumption, 10 to 20 percent butane or propane propellant, up to 5 percent acrylic hair stiffener, and a 5–15 percent mix of other chemicals. The term *Ocean* is derived from the oceanlike foam that is generated when the hair spray is mixed with water and rapidly shaken to release the butane or propane propellant.) The NCI study, which examined Ocean use by 178 males and 47 females, found that 10 percent of people ingesting Ocean were experimental users, that 50 percent drank Ocean to cure or alleviate alcohol hangover, and that 40 percent were chronic users who used Ocean daily for intoxication. (The onset of Ocean euphoria is rapid in comparison to that of other liquor, and chronic users almost always enter a blackout level of consciousness.) The study also revealed that 40 percent of Ocean users were experiencing medical complications that began after their initial use of it. Warning that teenage use of Ocean was potentially explosive, the NCI researchers recommended that state legislation to limit access to hair spray be enacted, and that programs for retailer awareness and public awareness, as well as prevention and education programs for children and young people, be undertaken.[32]

The Robert Wood Johnson Foundation's Healthy Nations Program

When funding for Northwest New Mexico Fighting Back came to an end in the spring of 1997, Daw and his colleagues applied for and received a $930,000, three-year grant to participate in a Robert Wood Johnson Foundation program called Healthy Nations: Reducing Substance Abuse Among Native Americans. This program had begun in early 1994, when the Foundation started financing fifteen tribes and Native American organizations for initiatives designed to combat alcoholism and substance abuse by addressing contributory problems, such as a deteriorating sense of cultural heritage; lack of consistent opposition to substance abuse within individual communities; and strong peer pressure among Native

American youths to drink, smoke, and use illegal drugs. The drastic need for programs to reduce alcohol and substance abuse among Native American youths can be seen in a risk behavior survey that was conducted in early 1998 in twenty-two of twenty-four Navajo Nation high schools, with 4,069 out of 6,250 eligible students participating. Nearly one-third of all students reported heavy binge drinking (five or more drinks of alcohol in a row) during the previous thirty days, almost two-thirds of all students reported using marijuana, and nearly 16 percent reported having used cocaine.[33]

In their grant application to The Robert Wood Johnson Foundation's Healthy Nations Program, Daw and his coworkers pointed out that during the previous five years Northwest New Mexico Fighting Back had successfully engaged all tribes, municipalities, and alcohol and drug service providers in the tricounty area in northwestern New Mexico, and that as a result of strong community support and response, there had been a significant reduction in alcohol and drug-related deaths. However, they went on to point out that the region still ranked high in alcohol-related homicide, crime, fatalities, and car crashes. As a result, they proposed programs to promote public awareness, foster intercultural relations, and improve treatment and prevention services for alcohol and substance abusers in six target areas, with a Healthy Nations coordinator assigned to each of them. The target areas included all villages in the pueblos of Acoma and Laguna; the Navajo chapter communities of Shiprock, Sanostee, Burnham, Sheep Springs, Newcomb, and Naschitti; the chapter communities of Counselor, Nageezi, Huerfano, Ojo, Encino, and Puerto Pintado; the chapter communities of Crownpoint, Marino Lake, Smith Lake, Pinedale, and Becenti; and the chapter communities of Tohatchi, Crystal, Mexican Springs, Navajo, and Window Rock.[34] (Readers of Tony Hillerman novels will no doubt remember his Navajo police heroes, Officer Jim Chee and Lt. Joe Leaphorn, driving to and from many of these communities.)

Dennis Lorenzo, a fifty-year-old Acoma who is director of the aftercare program at the Na'nizhoozhi Center, also served as the Healthy Nations coordinator for the Acoma pueblo. As he reported recently:

> The transition from Fighting Back to Healthy Nations was relatively smooth
> because the goals of both programs were essentially the same, and because Fight-
> ing Back had already developed education and treatment programs in several of
> the target areas. In the Acoma pueblo, a community action team organized an

"Earth Day" celebration during which 120 trees were planted. As part of the celebration, many Acoma families participated in traditional healing ceremonies. The action team also held community forums on how to prevent and deal with alcohol and substance abuse. In coordination with Acoma Behavioral Health Services, the team brought public attention to the problem posed by the sale of alcoholic beverages at a Wal-Mart in Cibola County. In addition, forums were held to foster stronger awareness of diabetes—a disease that had become a major health problem in the pueblo—and to emphasize the need for healthier eating habits.

In the six other target areas, action teams and volunteer groups carried out similar initiatives. The Tohatchi Healthy Nations Program organized six weeks of summer sports activities and camps, including a Little League in which 175 youths participated. Tohatchi also established a youth center and a Police Athletic League. Crownpoint's special focus was development of a community coalition to meet the needs of youth with workshops and Gathering of Native Americans' events. The coalition organized a policing project to reduce substance abuse and violence within several local housing projects and helped start a ROPES (Realization of Personal Excellence and Strength) program as well as a youth athletic association. The Healthy Nations coordinator at Crownpoint established a referral network for alcohol abusers with the Na'nizhoozhi Center and the Crownpoint Department of Behavioral Health Services. A family harmony program in the Crownpoint target area established a toll-free number for victims of domestic abuse.[35]

Early in the Healthy Nations Program, the community coalition at Counselor brought about the thirty-day suspension of a local bar license. During that time, public drunkenness decreased significantly, and there were no alcohol-related motor vehicle accidents in the community. Subsequently, the Counselor coalition was able to close down three of the four liquor retailers in the surrounding area. The coalition also cosponsored the annual Red Ribbon Memorial March and Gathering along eighty miles of New Mexico State Highway 44, where numerous alcohol-related traffic accidents and deaths had occurred. In the Shiprock area, the annual Joey Harry Memorial Run was held to honor the memory of Joey Harry, a seven-year-old girl who was killed by a drunken driver in 1995 in Newcomb, a remote community midway along the ninety-mile stretch of U.S. Highway 666 that runs north from Gallup to Shiprock.[36] A highlight of the

Healthy Nations effort in Shiprock was the signing of an intergovernmental agreement to create the Navajo Nation-Farmington Substance Abuse Task Force. (Farmington is a border town thirty miles east of Shiprock in the northwestern section of San Juan County.) The historic agreement included the Navajo Nation, San Juan County, and the City of Farmington and was cosigned by a dozen private providers of treatment and services for alcohol and substance abusers.[37]

In addition to supporting initiatives in the six target areas, the Healthy Nations program took the lead in organizing the annual Red Ribbon Multicultural Relay Run, an event dedicated to opposing alcohol and substance abuse in which five thousand runners from Native American and non-Native American communities across the state converge from three directions upon Albuquerque. (All of New Mexico's twenty-two Native American tribes were represented in the run.) In collaboration with the Na'nizhoozhi Center, the Healthy Nations program started off the new millennium with a Sobriety Pow-Wow at the University of New Mexico College in Gallup, which was attended by nearly seven hundred people. The program also organized a national healing conference for Native American adult children of alcoholics, which was attended by more than one hundred people, some of whom have since taken the lead in persuading the Navajo Nation to enhance its anti-bootlegging laws by increasing fines and jail time for offenders.

—w— The Future: Expanding to Other Towns Bordering the Navajo Reservation

Although many of the programs in the target areas have continued since Robert Wood Johnson Foundation funding for Healthy Nations ended in the summer of 2000, scores of Navajo and other Native American communities still need help to combat alcohol and substance abuse. For example, many of the 110 Navajo communities don't have service providers to assist them in this fight. From the very beginning, planners of Northwest New Mexico Fighting Back realized that their most daunting task was to offer education, treatment, and prevention programs for a large and culturally diverse population whose members were scattered over a vast rural area under the jurisdiction of no less than fourteen governmental agencies (including those of federal, state, county, and city governments and of four sovereign Native American nations). In their 1991

Implementation Plan, they recognized that the region affected by alcohol and substance abuse was far greater than the tricounty area targeted by the Fighting Back program, and they wondered if it should be enlarged to include parts of Arizona and Utah.[38] In this connection, they discussed the need for a "regional substance abuse authority," but because of the complex sovereignty issues involved they were not able to conceptualize, let alone establish, one. This was a failing that hindered alcohol reform in the Navajo Nation for most of the next decade.

In early June 2000, the Navajo Nation sponsored a two-day Behavioral Health Summit at the Civic Center in Farmington. The conference was attended by more than four hundred behavioral health specialists, physicians, and concerned citizens from the huge Four Corners Region that surrounds the point at which the borders of New Mexico, Arizona, Utah, and Colorado come together. In his opening remarks, Kelsey A. Begaye, president of the Navajo Nation, reminded his listeners that alcoholism had been the "scourge of the Navajo people for as long as we can remember," and a major contributor to motor vehicle fatalities, domestic violence, child abuse, elder abuse, acute mental illness, and other severe health problems. He called for a new and far broader initiative to be directed toward correcting the fragmentation and lack of coordination among the numerous federal, state, county, city, tribal, and private organizations that provide behavioral health services to the Navajo people and their neighbors living in towns bordering the reservation, and he announced the formation of a task force that would establish a behavioral health entity with sufficient credibility and authority to enable the Navajo Nation and its non-Navajo partners to efficiently combat the problem of alcohol and substance abuse in the Four Corners region.

A year and a half later, an organization called the Navajo Nation Regional Behavioral Health Consortium is being organized. The consortium will be made up of tribal and city governments in the Four Corners Region and include the mayors of Flagstaff, Farmington, Gallup, and eleven other cities in the area. (Federal, state, county, and private behavioral health agencies will act in an advisory capacity.) The mission of the consortium is to provide a comprehensive, high-quality behavioral health service delivery system to the residents of the region by coordinating the resources of its members. Start-up money will come from the tribes and the cities, which will seek an annual operating budget of some

$650,000 from the federal government. Among the problems that remained to be worked out at the beginning of 2002 were exchange of memoranda of understanding between the consortium and federal, state, county, city, and tribal health resource organizations; articles of incorporation and bylaws; establishment of a regional regulatory office to assist in licensing behavioral health facilities and providers; a method of developing behavioral health services to provide training in skills that will enable clients to support themselves; and identifying the availability and accessibility of culturally appropriate regional behavioral health services, such as detoxification, outpatient and inpatient programs, and aftercare support for children, adolescents, and adults.

Just how desperately the Navajo Nation needs this new initiative can be seen in a recent study on mortality trends in McKinley County that was conducted for Northwest New Mexico Fighting Back by Bernard Ellis & Associates. A report of the study, which was issued in August 2001, shows that the earlier pace of improvement in alcohol and substance-abuse-related accidents and deaths has slowed since 1995, and that in some cases the situation is worsening. For example, during the four-year period from 1995 to 1999, alcohol-induced mortality in McKinley County rose by 28 percent, drug-induced mortality increased by 135 percent, and suicide mortality increased by 58 percent. As a result, the Ellis & Associates report declared, "It is critically important that a renewed effort be initiated if progress toward reducing substance abuse in McKinley County is to continue."[39]

With this adjuration in mind, it can only be hoped that the newly formed consortium will prove to be an effective impetus in the long and difficult journey toward alcohol reform that has been under way in the Navajo Nation for more than a decade.

Notes

1. "Gallup: Paved With Good Intentions," *Albuquerque Tribune*, 28 September 1988, pp. A-1, Editorial, A-7.
2. Guthrie, P. *Case Histories in Alcohol Policy*. Trauma Foundation, 1999a, p. 146.
3. Gomez, D., and Guthrie, P. "Freebies Let Drunks Soak Up Another Day," *Albuquerque Tribune*, 28 September 1988, pp. A-3, A-10.

4. Guthrie, P., "A Family Outpouring," Albuquerque Tribune, 27 September 1988, p. A-3.
5. Editorial, *Albuquerque Tribune*, 27 September 1988, p. A-7.
6. "Gallup: Paved with Good Intentions," *Albuquerque Tribune*, 28 September 1988, p. A-1.
7. Robert Wood Johnson Foundation, *Grant Description for Fighting Back Project*, Jan. 29, 1990, p. 12–13.
8. Bernard Ellis & Associates. "Executive Summary: Alcohol Reform in Indian Country," April 7, 2000, Santa Fe, Tennessee.
9. Guthrie (1999a), p. 146.
10. Gomez, D., and Guthrie, P. "Freebies Let Drunks Soak Up Another Day," *Albuquerque Tribune,* 28 September 1988, p. A-5.
11. Gomez, D. "She Died with a Beer Can in Her Hand," *Albuquerque Tribune*, 29 September 1988, p. A-6.
12. "Gallup: The Killing Season," *Albuquerque Tribune*, 26 September 1988, p. A-1.
13. "Gallup: Six-pack to Go," *Albuquerque Tribune,* 29 September 1988, p. A-1.
14. Editorial, *Albuquerque Tribune*, 29 September 1988, p. A-9.
15. *Grant Description . . .* (1990), p. 16
16. *Grant Description . . .* (1990), pp. 13–14.
17. "Gallup: The Town Drunk," *Albuquerque Tribune*, 1 October 1988, p. A-1
18. *Grant Description . . .* (1990), p. 13.
19. Guthrie, P. "Gallup, New Mexico: On the Road to Recovery." *In Case Histories . . .* (1999b), p. 150.
20. Guthrie (1999b), p. 151.
21 Guthrie, P. "A Family Outpouring," *Albuquerque Tribune*, 27 September 1988, p. A-5.
22. Guthrie, P., and Gomez, D. "Year In, Year Out, the Same Story," *Albuquerque Tribune*, 1 October 1988, p. A-5.
23. Haederle, M. "American Album: 'Drunk City' Faces up to its Sobering Problems," *Los Angeles Times*, 14 May 1990, p. A-5.
24. Gomez, D. "Family Ministering to Indians Cut in Half by Drunk Driver," *Albuquerque Tribune*, 8 February 1999, D-1.
25. Guthrie (1999b), p. 153.
26. Guthrie (1999b), p. 156.

27. Northwest New Mexico Council of Governments. *Implementation Proposal for the Fighting Back Initiative.* Sept. 9, 1991, p.19.

28. *Implementation Proposal . . .* (1991), Part 1, p. 11.

29. *Implementation Proposal . . .* (1991), Project Management Section, p.2.

30. Bernard Ellis & Associates. "Taking the Long View." Sept. 28, 1994, Santa Fe, Tennessee.

31. Bernard Ellis & Associates. "A Longer View." Jan. 10, 1997, Santa Fe, Tennessee.

32. *"Ocean" Awareness Project Report.* Na'Nizhoozhi Center, 1999, p. 10.

33. *Youth Risk Behavior Survey.* Navajo Nation High Schools. Feb. 6, 1998, pp. 10, 11.

34. Northwest New Mexico Fighting Back. *First Annual Narrative Report for Healthy Nations Grant.* Dec. 21, 1998, pp. 1–14.

35. Northwest Next Mexico Fighting Back. Annual Narrative Progress Report for July 98–July 99. Aug. 26, 1999, pp. 1–12.

36. Northwest New Mexico Fighting Back. Final Narrative Progress Report for July 1997 Through June 200. Oct. 17, 2000, pp. 1–14.

37. Implementation Proposal . . . (1991), Objectives Section, p. 9.

38. Implementation Proposal . . . (1991), Section on Collaboration and Cooperation, p. 2.

39. Bernard Ellis & Associates. "The Long and the Short View." Aug. 27, 2001, pp. 1–31.

Strengthening Human Capacity

8

Building Health Policy Research Capacity in the Social Sciences

David C. Colby

Editors' Introduction

Foundations are often criticized for focusing on the quick hit—a project that has the potential for a visible impact in the short run. Yet meaningful change often comes about through strategies that have a longer-term focus and whose results are not immediately visible. Although The Robert Wood Johnson Foundation is not immune from pursuing the quick hit, it has also had the patience and endurance to adopt strategies that seek longer-term results. One example is its investment in building the quality of the health workforce. From its earliest days, the Foundation devoted a substantial share of its resources to improving the health workforce, including nurses, physicians, policy experts, medical school faculty members, and researchers. Currently, education and training grants represent 18 percent of the Foundation's portfolio of commitments.

Strengthening the health workforce has been a recurring topic in *The Robert Wood Johnson Foundation Anthology* series. The first *Anthology* included a chapter analyzing the overall logic and history of investments in workforce programs.[1] The 1998–99 *Anthology* contained a chapter on the Foundation's investments in training for nurse practitioners and physician assistants,[2] the 2000 *Anthology* highlighted the workings of the Minority Medical Education Program,[3] and last year's volume discussed the Health Policy Fellows Program.[4]

This chapter, written by David C. Colby, a senior program officer at The Robert Wood Johnson Foundation, examines the Foundation's investments in building capacity among social scientists to do health policy analysis. The series of programs analyzed by Colby underscores the Foundation's commitment to building health policy expertise among social science researchers at the nation's academic institutions. Colby traces the evolution of the Foundation's programs from its initial support of four well-established university professors; through an unsuccessful fellowship program in health care finance; to its two current, more tightly structured fellowship programs.

Interest in workforce initiatives remains strong at The Robert Wood Johnson Foundation—so strong, in fact, that these initiatives are considered to be "core" programs. In October 2001, the board approved a multi-year renewal and reshaping of the Clinical Scholars Program, and in April 2002, it approved initiation of a new Health and Society Scholars Program.

1. Isaacs, S. L., Sandy, L. G., and Schroeder, S. A. "Improving the Health Care Workforce: Perspectives from Twenty-Four Years' Experience." In *To Improve Health and Health Care 1997: The Robert Wood Johnson Foundation Anthology.* San Francisco: Jossey-Bass, 1997.
2. Keenan, T. "Support of Nurse-Practitioners and Physician Assistants." In *To Improve Health and Health Care 1998–1999: The Robert Wood Johnson Foundation Anthology.* San Francisco: Jossey-Bass, 1998.
3. Bergeisen, L., and Cantor, J. "The Minority Medical Education Program." In *To Improve Health and Health Care 2000: The Robert Wood Johnson Foundation Anthology.* San Francisco: Jossey-Bass, 2000.
4. Frank, R. "The Health Policy Fellowship Program." In *To Improve Health and Health Care, Vol. V. The Robert Wood Johnson Foundation Anthology,* San Francisco: Jossey-Bass, 2002.

—*w*— $\mathbf{T}$he Robert Wood Johnson Foundation has devoted far more of its resources to moving health professionals into health policy research and health services research than to attracting social scientists to these fields. From its beginnings in 1972, the Foundation recognized the need to train physicians to address health policy, access, financing, and related issues. In 1972, the Foundation took over the Clinical Scholars program from the Commonwealth Fund and the Carnegie Corporation and expanded it substantially. This program trains physicians in the social sciences, especially in the research methods of the social science disciplines. In 1973, the Foundation created the Health Policy Fellowships program, which introduces physicians and other midcareer health professionals to federal policy making. These are the Foundation's two longest-running programs.

In contrast, the Foundation's attempts to bring social scientists into health policy analysis and research developed more slowly. It first awarded grants to two research institutions to teach and conduct research on health policy, especially health economics. The Foundation next gave awards to a small number of highly regarded university professors (the so-called "great men awards") to support their research in health policy and health services. Over the years, the great men awards evolved into a fellowship program called Investigator Awards in Health Policy Research. A companion fellowship program, Scholars in Health Policy Research, was established to bring economists, political scientists, and sociologists into health policy research. Both of these fellowship programs are still in existence. The goal of these two programs—and a third one, the Faculty Fellowships in Health Care Finance, which the Foundation funded in the 1980s—has been to attract social scientists to health policy analysis and health services research and to maintain their commitment to these fields.

The author thanks Alan Cohen and Terrance Keenan for their helpful comments on earlier versions of this chapter and Ayorkor Gaba for her research assistance.

—ɯ— Early Efforts: 1972 to 1987

During the Foundation's first fifteen years, its commitment to attracting social scientists to health policy research was minimal and its efforts were not strategic. Social scientists themselves were slow to take to the health policy field. Even though the passage of Medicare and Medicaid in 1965 revealed the need for health policy research, social scientists entered this field only gradually over the next two decades. Discipline-based health policy journals were established in 1976 (*The Journal of Health Politics, Policy and Law*) and 1982 (*The Journal of Health Economics*). *Health Affairs,* the leading health policy journal, was founded with a grant from The Robert Wood Johnson Foundation in 1981. The Association for Health Services Research, whose membership includes both social scientists and health professionals, was also established in 1981.

In 1972, when the trustees considered priorities for the Foundation, they assumed that financing health care would be solved within three years with universal health insurance—a reasonable assumption, given the support of President Richard M. Nixon for a national health plan. The Nixon plan was one of several competing health insurance bills introduced at that time. One approach favored comprehensive national health insurance financed through the tax system; another called for income-related tax credits to encourage purchasing private insurance. But health care financing reform became a victim of Watergate and of political positioning for the 1974 congressional elections.

Regardless of the status of health reform, in the Foundation's first year the trustees set three goals:

1. Improving access for the underserved
2. Improving quality of care
3. Developing mechanisms for objective analysis of public policies (in 1975, this was changed to "encouraging the development of timely well-targeted policy research.")

At a meeting of the Foundation's board in January 1973, the trustees considered how to implement the last of the three goals and established the early research and policy agenda.

Health Policy Research and Health Economics Training

As an early priority, The Robert Wood Johnson Foundation wanted to develop independent, objective, applied policy centers; train individuals in policy analysis; and disseminate policy-relevant information in a useful form. In 1973, the Foundation funded a health policy research and teaching center at the University of California, San Francisco, led by Philip Lee, a physician who had been the assistant secretary for health in the Johnson administration. In addition to offering regular courses, the Health Policy Center established summer fellowships that gave graduate and professional students the opportunity to conduct research and participate in a health policy seminar; it also awarded predoctoral fellowships that offered the opportunity to work in health policy. The successor to the Health Policy Center, now known as the Institute for Health Policy Studies, remains active in health research and policy analysis.

Continuing a program begun by the Carnegie Corporation, The Robert Wood Johnson Foundation provided a three-year grant (1973–1976) to Harvard University to award doctoral and postdoctoral fellowships in health economics. Leading Harvard economists Martin Feldstein, Rashi Fein, and John Dunlop supervised the fellows. The results of these grants from Carnegie and Robert Wood Johnson were spectacular. The fellows included luminaries of the next generation of health economists, such as Harold Luft, William Hsiao, William White, Paul Ginsburg, and David Salkever. Nevertheless, Harvard returned much of the money, finding that many young economists hesitated to choose health as their specialty field.

The "Great Men Awards"

To reach its goal of "developing mechanisms for objective analysis of public policies," the Foundation provided funding, over a number of years, for the policy analysis and research of a few well-established outstanding scholars. These grants were awarded under permissive ground rules unlike those for most research efforts. Commenting on one of the grants in 1976, a Foundation staff member wrote a memo to the board of trustees, stating that "a small amount of Foundation support of scholars . . . helps to underwrite a type of creativity not possible with our highly targeted research studies and calls our attention to a range of possible fields of interest in the health sector that our normal program activities would not pick up."

Victor Fuchs   The first of these awards went to Victor Fuchs, who received four grants from 1973 to 1988. At the time of the first grant, Fuchs was a highly respected labor economist in his late forties. He was vice president of the National Bureau of Economic Research, a professor of community medicine at the Mount Sinai School of Medicine, a professor of economics at the City College of New York Graduate Center, and a member of the Institute of Medicine.

Fuchs's research interests, pursued under the four grants, were broad ranging. During the first grant, he conducted research on economic measurement of health. The second grant allowed him to focus on child health and pediatric care, adult health and health practices, the cost of medical care, training and utilization of allied health manpower, and the role of medical care and national health insurance in society. With the third grant, he developed measures of productivity and improvements in productivity in the health field. The fourth grant enabled Fuchs to focus on the health of the American people and on improving health markets. The grants also provided funds for training fellowships. By 1984, Fuchs had trained thirty-five economists and physicians, including Kenneth Warner, an economist who is now a leading expert on tobacco policy, and Alan Garber, at the time a medical student, who later received his Ph.D. in economics and his M.D. degree and became a leading health services researcher at Stanford University.

With support from The Robert Wood Johnson Foundation, Fuchs published three books—*Economic Aspects of Health* in 1982, *How We Live* in 1983, and *The Health Economy* in 1986—as well as numerous articles. His contributions to understanding medical care are widely known. Several of his other enduring contributions, however, are less appreciated. First, he applied economic concepts to people's lives, thereby demonstrating how difficult it is to understand health without understanding other aspects of life. Second, he shifted the focus of health economics from studies on medical care to those on health, thus pointing the way to investigating the social determinants of health.

David Mechanic   David Mechanic received three grants, providing support for research in the organization of health care services, which he conducted between 1973 and 1987. Unlike the other great men awards, Mechanic's first grant was shared with another faculty member at the University of Wisconsin.

In his thirties at the time of the initial grant, Mechanic was already a leading medical sociologist. He was the chairman of the sociology department and head of the Center for Medical Sociology and Health Services Research at the University of Wisconsin. Like Victor Fuchs, he was a member of the Institute of Medicine.

Mechanic's work encompassed the sociology of medicine, mental health, patient behavior, and the organization of ambulatory care. His ability to spot trends and research issues in their earliest stages was remarkable. He was one of the first researchers to recognize significant changes occurring in the medical care system, especially those involving managed care. Even when medical care spending was only 8.6 percent of the gross national product, he argued that cost containment would be an issue in the future.

In addition to supporting Mechanic's research, the Foundation's grants funded a number of predoctoral and postdoctoral fellowships under his tutelage. One of those fellows, Linda Aiken, subsequently served as a vice president of The Robert Wood Johnson Foundation and became a leading health service researcher at the University of Pennsylvania.

Eli Ginzberg   Eli Ginzberg received six grants, funding his research from 1973 to 1990. At the time of his first grant, Ginzberg was an economist in the Graduate School of Business at Columbia University. He was in his sixties and had already written forty books. He, too, had been elected a member of the Institute of Medicine.

With funding from the Foundation, Ginzberg and his colleagues produced important insights into health workforce issues. (Unlike the other recipients of these early awards, Ginzberg worked with a team of senior researchers.) In the mid-1970s, for example, he foresaw a surplus of physicians and nurses; yet, according to him, the surplus would not solve the problem of maldistribution of health care personnel or the problem of access to care. The long-term impact of his work, however, is probably in two other areas. First, his publication of *Changing U.S. Health Care: A Study of Four Metropolitan Areas* was a precursor of the Foundation's later investments to track changes in the American health care system. Second, over many years and in numerous places, he concluded that health reform can and probably should be done only incrementally.

William Schwartz   William Schwartz received four grants from 1976 to 1989. At the time of his first grant, he was the fifty-three-year-old chairman of the Department of Medicine at Tufts, physician-in-chief of the New England Medical Center, and a researcher with the RAND Corporation. He held the first endowed chair of medicine at Tufts and was a member of the Institute of Medicine.

The support from The Robert Wood Johnson Foundation allowed Schwartz to work on a broad range of national health problems, especially at the intersection of medicine and economics. He published leading articles (generally for a medical audience) on health care costs, physician supply, and malpractice. He concluded that expansion of the supply of physicians was one factor that accounted for increases in costs, along with demographic factors and greater insurance coverage. He argued that consolidation of hospital facilities, a popular policy solution at the time, would not reduce costs. Although his articles attracted considerable attention, his book *The Painful Prescription*, written with economist Henry Aaron, garnered the most attention. Schwartz and Aaron asked why Great Britain spends about half of what the United States does on hospital care per person. After examining the British system, where health care is rationed and expenditures are limited by reduced quantity, not quality, of care, they concluded that it would be more difficult to control costs in the United States than in Britain.

Assessment   The scholars receiving the great men awards were extremely productive. Their research was creative, and in many cases enduring. Nevertheless, the Foundation ran very little risk. It made bets on known winners. With the exception of David Mechanic, these awards were to scholars in their late forties, fifties, and sixties.

The grants were not open to all in a fair competition, and in 1987 the Foundation staff decided to stop renewing them and instead develop a program that would draw on the flexibility of the great men approach but be open to a greater number and variety of researchers. Several years later, this would be institutionalized as the Investigator Awards in Health Policy Research program.

Although it was not a central focus, some of the great men awards also funded training of younger scholars. As a result, a group of economists and physicians were trained in health economics. But the size of this effort was limited and had little impact on other social science disciplines. These efforts would be expanded and institutionalized first in the Faculty Fellows in Health Care Finance program and then in the Scholars in Health Policy Research program.

—ᴍ— Focusing on Cost Containment: 1984 to 1992

During the 1980s, the rising cost of health care became a nationally recognized concern. In an effort to slow down the spiraling costs, policy makers tried a number of measures. The most important was a change in how hospital costs were paid under Medicare, with the legislation in 1983 of "diagnostic-related groups." Health care finance became an important subdiscipline, and the Foundation, concerned that not enough scholars were gravitating toward it, felt there was a need to train faculty members to teach health finance in public health, management, and related schools. The Foundation hoped to produce leaders in health care finance whose stature would rival the alumni of the Clinical Scholars program.

The Faculty Fellowships in Health Care Finance Program

The Faculty Fellowships in Health Care Finance began in 1984 and continued through 1992. The program extended a three-part opportunity to six fellows per year. In the first year, the fellows were introduced to the latest developments in health care finance through an intensive three-month (later a four-month) educational program at Johns Hopkins University. This was followed by a nine-month (later an eight-month) placement in a public or private health care financing organization. During the second year, the fellows returned to their university positions, receiving up to $15,000 to conduct research on health care finance. Forty fellows went through the program.

Two former fellows are examples of the kind of people recruited and their subsequent careers. At the time of entering the fellowship in 1984, Kyle Grazier had received a doctorate in public health from the University of California, Berkeley, had been awarded a Kellogg Fellowship in Health Care Finance, had published articles on cost accounting and reimbursement issues, and was assistant professor in the School of Medicine at Yale University. Since leaving the program, she has taught courses in health and corporate finance, insurance, and management topics as a faculty member at Yale, the University of California, Berkeley, Cornell, and the University of Michigan. She has published articles on reimbursement systems, behavioral health, managed care, accounting, and insurance.

Mark Hall, an attorney with a law degree from the University of Chicago, had published a limited amount on the legal issues related to cost containment and was a law professor at Arizona State University before his fellowship. After leaving the program, he returned to Arizona State and later took a position in the law school at Wake Forest University. He has published on health care law, rationing, genetics and insurance, and physician incentives. Probably his most important work in health care financing has been on health insurance market reforms.

Despite some individual successes, an outside evaluation team and the Foundation staff judged the Faculty Fellowships program to be a failure.[1] They found that there was little agreement between the National Program Office, Foundation staff, and the fellows on the purpose of the program, nor even on the definition of health care finance. The disagreement obviously affected the program. First, the type of fellow to be recruited was unclear. For example, was the program to enhance the knowledge of professors of health care finance, or to train faculty members from, say, economics or public policy in health financing? Second, because the focus of the program was not clearly defined, the curriculum itself was never in proper focus. It was not clear, for example, whether the fellows should be learning accounting and management or whether they should be learning health care financing. Although the Foundation initially may have had the former in mind, the leaders of the program at the Johns Hopkins School of Hygiene and Public Health, first Carl Schramm and later Susan Horn, were more interested in the latter.

The program's impact was marginal. With a few exceptions, it neither recruited nor developed many future academic stars in the fields of health care finance and policy. Nearly ten years after the program closed, even though nearly three-fourths of the former fellows are in the health care field only two are teaching health care finance.

This program may have been misguided. If the Foundation had the narrow goal of training those already in the field of health care finance, the number of eligible faculty members was quite small. Moreover, the fellows recruited from the liberal arts, such as economists and political scientists, had difficulty returning to their departments. Additionally, a one-size-fits-all curriculum at a single institution did not meet the needs of fellows with varied backgrounds.

—ᴠᴠ— Strengthening the Health Policy Research Workforce: 1992 to the Present

With funding for a small number of great men awards having ended and the Faculty Fellowships in Health Care Finance program winding down, the Foundation reconsidered how best to attract gifted social scientists to health policy analysis and health services research. Steven Schroeder, president of the Foundation, was concerned that broad policy thinkers such as Victor Fuchs had been replaced by narrow methodologists, especially among economists. In 1992, the Foundation embarked on a new strategy by funding two related programs. The first, the Scholars in Health Policy Research Program, aimed at attracting young economists, political scientists, and sociologists to careers in health policy research, thus building a core of experts from these three disciplines. The second, the Investigator Awards in Health Policy Research Program, funded innovative research ideas proposed by researchers—both rising and established—from a variety of disciplines.

Scholars in Health Policy Research (1992 to the Present)

Scholars in Health Policy Research is a two-year fellowship program designed to attract top economists, political scientists, and sociologists early in their careers to health policy by improving their knowledge of health policy, providing them with mentoring from senior faculty members, and encouraging them to conduct health policy research. The program represents institutionalization of the earlier, mostly informal Foundation attempts at building capacity in the social sciences.

The National Advisory Committee for this program has been a key factor in its development. Although the committee's membership has changed over time, it has typically had twelve to fourteen members, among them sociologists, political scientists, and economists. Most of the members have conducted health research, although others have done research only in related fields. About half of the advisory committee members hold faculty appointments in a social science discipline. The others come from schools of medicine, public health, business, and public policy. The stature of the committee members helps to attract applicants to the program. The committee members participate in selecting scholars, assist the National Program Office in conducting site visits, and help mentor individual scholars.

Three academic sites housing the scholars were chosen from universities that had a top department in economics, political science, or sociology plus a top school of medicine or public health. Yale University, the University of Michigan, and the combination of the University of California, Berkeley, and the University of California, San Francisco were selected as the original sites. The geographic diversity of the sites, their curricula, and the varying interests and strengths of the faculty attracted different scholars to the sites.[2] If the Scholars in Health Policy Research program had established only one site, as did the Faculty Fellowships in Health Care Finance program, it would have had limited opportunities and probably would not have attracted as broad-based a group of scholars as it has.

Originally, applicants were to be selected from the three disciplines (economics, political science, and sociology) and to have received their doctoral degrees within the previous three years. These requirements have been modified over the years. Even though nearly all of the Scholars come from the field of sociology, political science, or economics, there have been exceptions. The program has accepted a few Scholars who received a degree in a related field, such as public policy or history, and who also have demonstrated competence in one of the three disciplines. Additionally, very early in the program, it became apparent that the requirement that candidates have received their doctorates within the three previous years was too limiting. In 1997, the window was widened to five years.

Learning from the Faculty Fellowships in Health Care Finance program, the Scholars in Health Policy Research program recruits potential applicants more aggressively and in a more personal fashion. In addition to the usual call for applications and notices placed in newsletters of the three disciplinary national associations, the National Program Office sends letters to the chairs and placement officers of top departments in each discipline. Recruitment events, in which faculty members from the sites, National Advisory Committee members, and Scholars participate, are held at the annual meeting of each discipline's national association. In addition, there are intensive efforts, including special mailings, to recruit minority scholars.

Recruiting top economists has proven more difficult than recruitment in the two other disciplines for several reasons. The salaries of academic economists are higher than those of the two other disciplines. Also, economists do not have much experience with postdoctoral fellowships. This difficulty in recruiting economists was surprising, given the Foundation's early success with economists in the Harvard fellowship program and the feeling of some senior Foundation staff members that economists would be the most important scholars to recruit.

Recruiting political scientists has been easier. A breakthrough occurred when Richard Hall, a leading congressional scholar at the University of Michigan, wanted to recruit strong political scientists to the Michigan Scholars program. He called leading political scientists about their best current or recent graduate students and then sent personal letters to these graduate students or new faculty members; he followed up with phone calls. Most political scientists would not have identified this program as an opportunity to advance their careers, but the personalization of the recruitment heightened awareness of the program, selling it with political scientists. Recruitment of sociologists has been harder than that of political scientists, but easier than that of economists.

The Scholars in Health Policy Research program typically receives about one hundred applications a year. The National Program Office, which is located at Boston University's School of Management and directed by Alan Cohen, screens them and selects about half for review by the National Advisory Committee. The Committee winnows the list to about twenty-five finalists. They are interviewed on campus at the sites. In a matching process, the sites and the finalists rank their selections. On the basis of the rankings, the National Program Office and the Foundation match scholars and sites. The process is designed to produce a balance of disciplines at each site, and to honor the first choices of sites and scholars whenever possible. Approximately twelve scholars are selected each year. At the end of 2001, the program had selected ninety-five scholars: twenty-seven economists, thirty-seven political scientists, and thirty-one sociologists. There were fifty-eight men and thirty-seven women. Eleven of the Scholars were members of a minority; most were selected in the later years of the program.

One difficult issue in the selection is how much weight to place on an applicant's prior knowledge of and involvement in health and health policy. Those with related interests, for example in welfare policy or labor economics, are very attractive to the program; their knowledge base is relevant, and the value added by the program is clear. Those with a prior degree in public health are usually not selected, because the value added by the program is judged to be limited. Between these extremes—for example, a person who has written one or two papers on a health-related topic—it is a judgment call about how much value the program will add to the person's career in health policy research.

During their two years in the program, the Scholars in Health Policy Research participate in a range of activities. They take an introductory course or seminar on health and health policy, as well as research seminars with presentations by the Scholars themselves and by outside speakers. They are given time, funding, and other resources to conduct research. The Scholars participate in seminars in their home discipline. They also have one or two senior faculty mentors who offer career advice, work on joint research projects, and help in the search for a job.

Originally, the Scholars in Health Policy Research were given the opportunity to have a field placement in a Washington-based health policy organization, such as the Health Care Financing Administration, the Physician Payment Review Commission, or the Office of Technology Assessment. As the program developed, however, both the Scholars and the senior faculty members at the three training sites felt that staying at the academic site for the full two years would be more beneficial. Thus, the field placement was dropped after the first two years, giving the program a more academic orientation.

The National Program Office holds an annual meeting for the Scholars in Health Policy Research; it is attended by the Scholars, faculty members from the sites, National Advisory Committee members, staff members from the national program offices of the Scholars in Health Policy Research and Investigator Awards in Health Policy Research programs, several Clinical Scholars, and Foundation staff members. At the annual meeting, first-year Scholars present their ideas for future research in an environment that allows them to gain knowledge, improve their methodology, and develop contacts; second-year Scholars present finished research.

To offer a forum for ongoing exchange of ideas and research, the National Program Office also sponsors a "working papers" series for the scholars and faculty associated with the program. By mid-2002, some twenty-three had appeared in this series.

The Scholars in Health Policy Research program has attracted top scholars and has changed the career trajectory of many of them. Paula Lantz, who received her Ph.D. in sociology from the University of Wisconsin and was in the first cohort of scholars at the University of Michigan from 1994 to 1996, is an example of one kind of scholar the program attracts. She is currently an associate professor of public health at the University of Michigan, conducting research on legal and illegal drugs, cancer treatments, and social determinants of health. The author of more than twenty-five peer-reviewed articles, numerous chapters in books and other publications, and a book, she is a member of the core faculty for the Clinical Scholars Program at the University of Michigan and the codirector of the Scholars in Health Policy Research Program there. She is an example of a Health Policy Research Scholar who was trained in a top-ranked department, who had an interest in health before joining the program, and whose career was given a boost by the program.

By contrast, Daniel Carpenter received his doctorate in political science from the University of Chicago in 1996, writing a dissertation on the federal agriculture, interior, and post office departments. The recipient of numerous awards before he entered the program, he was expected to be a political science star even before his acceptance as a Scholar. From 1998 to 2000, he was a Health Policy Research Scholar at the University of Michigan. In 2000, he won the best paper award at the Midwest Political Science Association Meeting for a paper on the political economy of the Food and Drug Administration's approval process. After leaving the program, he received a National Science Foundation grant to continue his work on the FDA. In his case, the program captured a strong discipline-based scholar who had shown no interest in health and redirected some of his interests toward health policy.

The program has also had another impact: enriching the intellectual life at the sites. Many faculty members became interested in health services and policy projects for the first time. For example, Richard Hall, the political scientist who recruited many Scholars in Health Policy Research, became interested in lobbying on health issues. Ian Shapiro, a faculty member at Yale, discussed health for the first time in his book, *Democratic Justice,* after being involved with the Scholars program.

The program appears to have had the greatest impact on political science. Even though political scientists had the least experience with health and health policy research, they seemed to appreciate this program and benefit from it more than Scholars from the fields of sociology and economics.

The Scholars program has had a number of issues to resolve. One is how to balance a Scholar's work in his or her home discipline and research in other disciplines. The program tried to strengthen Scholars' ties to their own social science discipline, while encouraging appreciation of the insights and methods of the other two disciplines. For recently educated scholars, strong disciplinary (or even subdisciplinary) ties are extremely important. They have spent the previous years immersed in the discipline, and career advancement is often based on doing research into questions of importance to their discipline. Thus, the Scholars and the sites have had to work to balance disciplinary depth and multidisciplinary breadth.

Another source of tension has been in the use of methodological approaches, especially between quantitative and qualitative research. Scholars often feel strongly about their methodological approaches. In the early years, the methodological issues were intertwined with disciplinary and gender differences. Economists have tended to be men with quantitative approaches, while sociologists have tended to be women with qualitative approaches. Political scientists have a mix of methodological approaches. The National Program Office fostered open discussion of the issue in a plenary session at the 1997 annual meeting, and sites have been encouraged to continue the dialogue about the issue.

As with the earlier Faculty Fellowships in Health Care Finance program, designing and teaching the introductory course on health issues has been difficult because the Scholars have such varying levels of knowledge. Additionally, as the program matured and actively sought individuals who were new to health, the Scholars were less likely to have expertise in health policy. In response, each site has redesigned the core curriculum.

In sum, the Scholars in Health Policy Research Program has attracted high-quality disciplinary scholars, changed the interests of some, reinforced the interests of others, strengthened the career opportunities of many, and broadened their understanding of health policy and the other disciplines. It has also stimulated the intellectual life, research, and teaching interests of faculty at the sites.

Investigator Awards in Health Policy Research (1992 to the Present)

In the early 1990s, as they were considering how to strengthen the health policy capacity of the social sciences, staff members at The Robert Wood Johnson Foundation concluded that the fields of health services research and health policy analysis had developed substantially but that the research was often too narrow. They also felt that too few senior scholars were doing health policy research. The Foundation decided that it needed to develop a program that encouraged health policy researchers to take risks and do innovative work like that done under the great men awards, but without the closed nature of the latter program. Thus, as part of the same strategy that developed the Scholars in Health Policy Research Program, the Foundation also developed the Investigator Awards in Health Policy Research Program. The purpose of the Investigator Awards program was to bolster top researchers in health policy and to attract new researchers, especially from the social sciences, to the field of health policy.

The Investigator Awards program supports creative, innovative health policy research projects, most of which would not be funded otherwise. From 1993 to 2001, the program provided grants of up to $250,000 for a three-year period. Currently, the award level is up to $275,000, and about ten awards are made each year.

The National Advisory Committee for the Investigator Award program consists of leading scholars (including some past Award recipients), usually representing a broad range of disciplines. In contrast to the National Advisory Committee for the Scholars in Health Policy Research program, the National Advisory Committee for the Investigator Awards program focuses mainly on selecting awardees.

It is a process that takes a relatively long time. To get the word out, the National Program Office, located at the Institute for Health, Health Care Policy, and Aging Research at Rutgers University and directed by David Mechanic, conducts formal recruitment meetings and supports panels for the presentation of Investigators' research at professional meetings. A formal call for applications is sent to a large list of scholars, mostly at universities, research organizations, and think tanks. In addition, advertisements and notices are placed in newsletters and journals, including those for minorities.

Applicants send a letter of intent to the National Program Office in the early spring. There have been between 181 and 503 letters of intent each year. The National Program Office director, National Advisory Committee members, and Foundation staff members review and rank the letters of intent, selecting about fifty finalists who are asked to submit a full proposal, which is due in the summer. The National Advisory Committee selects ten awardees in the late fall.

Through the end of 2001, more than three thousand candidates applied for an Investigator Award. From 1993 to 2001, the program awarded 83 grants to 103 individuals (awards are made to individuals, but in some cases two people jointly received an award). Although the early Investigators were about two-thirds men, in later years the gender balance has become relatively equal.[3] Nevertheless, the number of minority Investigators has been slim, with only five nonwhites winning awards.

The awards have been made to scholars from a broad range of disciplines, including economics, medicine, law, political science and public policy, sociology, history, health services research, and public health. Nevertheless, from 1993 to 2001, over half of the awards went to economists, sociologists, and political scientists.

The research funded under the Investigator Awards program has been broad in scope, and the methodology flexible. Nevertheless, unlike the great men awards—which were made to support individuals who were given great leeway in the research they carried out—these awards are made to fund research itself.

Several examples illustrate the range, the intellectual nature, and the flexibility of the research carried out under the Investigator Awards program. As a result of his award, David Smith, a professor in the business school at Temple University, published *Health Care Divided: Race and Healing a Nation.* In this historical study, he examined the link between previous racial segregation and discrimination today, described efforts to end discrimination in health care through the courts and federal regulation, and examined approaches to addressing continuing racial disparities in health and health care.

With his award, James Robinson, an economist at the University of California, Berkeley, wrote *The Corporate Practice of Medicine: Competition and Innovation in Health Care.* This book analyzes the transformation of medicine from a cottage industry with professional dominance to unmanaged competition with corporate dominance, turbulence, and creativity. Robinson's analysis indicates that the new health care organizations contain the seeds of their own destruction.

By contrast, Kenneth Warner, an economist at the University of Michigan who had earlier worked under Victor Fuchs at the National Bureau of Economic Research, chose a more applied topic. He had planned to write a book on the history of tobacco policy in the United States, but after he received the award, someone else published such a book. Nevertheless, with his award, he conducted research on tobacco policy that had a major impact. His editorials on the tobacco settlement in the *American Journal of Public Health* and *Tobacco Control* were so influential that he was invited to the White House to discuss the settlement with interested officials. His article on how to regulate the development and marketing of novel nicotine delivery devices in the *Journal of the American Medical Association* raised the consciousness of this problem among federal regulators and legislators.

The Investigator Awards program holds an annual meeting where newly selected Investigators can discuss their projects at an early stage and other Investigators can present finished projects. The formal parts of these meetings have been problematic, however, because they have been too packed with presentations. In addition to sharing knowledge through formal presentations, the value of the annual meeting lies in the informal contacts and networking, especially across disciplines.

Although the Investigators work individually on their research projects, an intellectual synergy can develop between Investigators working on the same general topic. To formalize this kind of exchange, the National Program Office supported cluster groups of Investigators working on similar topics. These groups have become important to the program. They have been formed on a number of topics:

- Social determinants of health
- Politics and health policy
- Transformation of the health care system
- Services for people with chronic conditions
- Health care institutions
- Trust and accountability
- Law and ethics
- Competition and regulation

Some cluster groups produced only a lively intellectual exchange, but others developed their own articles. As an example, the competition and regulation cluster group decided to examine Kenneth Arrow's seminal article, "Uncertainty and the Welfare Economics of Medical Care."[4] They analyzed how well Arrow's article described the situation in the early 1960s, how the health care market has changed, and how Arrow's concepts apply now. The project grew into a special issue of the *Journal of Health Politics, Policy and Law*—an issue that exemplifies the best of what can be done when individuals trained in multiple disciplines approach a problem.[5]

The Investigator Award has become prized not merely for the research money but also for its prestige. Those who have won the award have become more visible to the rest of the academic world and, to a lesser extent, the policy world. Although the projects are structured, they permit a great deal of freedom for a creative intellectual approach. As a whole, they have been intellectually exciting and have furthered understanding of the forces that shape the health care system and health policy.

—◊— Other Foundation Support of Social Science Research

The Robert Wood Johnson Foundation has also funded more targeted research of social scientists. From 1982 to 1987, the Foundation funded forty-four research projects under the Program for Demonstration and Research on Health Care Costs. In 1988, this program was expanded and became the Changes in Health Care Financing and Organization, or HCFO, program. By the end of 2001, the Foundation had authorized more than $50 million for grants under HCFO, funding 159 projects. More recently, the Foundation established the Substance Abuse Policy Research Program, authorizing $55 million for it since 1994. By January 2002, more than 160 projects were funded under this program. In addition, the Foundation has funded many individual research projects.

These research endeavors have no specific workforce goals, but they do provide funding for social scientists and others conducting health policy or health services research and give credibility to researchers selected under a prestigious program. Thus they have an indirect effect on the social science workforce.

—◊— Conclusions

Early in the Foundation's development, the leadership decided not to fund biomedical research because of the resources others were providing for such efforts. With the expectation that the passage of universal health insurance was near, the clinical, management, workforce, and policy challenges in delivering health care were seen as enormous and largely unaddressed. Thus, the Foundation chose to focus on social issues involved in health care. At that time, however, there was little interest in health even though the Foundation was dedicated to improving both the health and the health care of all Americans.

The Foundation had a slow start and much difficulty in developing programs to strengthen the health policy research capacity of the social science workforce. In many ways, this reflected the values and experiences of the leadership. The first three presidents of the Foundation came from academic medicine, and other leaders have had backgrounds in public health, nursing, and public policy. As a general rule, the leadership and staff have not been trained in the traditional social science disciplines.

The early efforts produced many creative research projects by giving a few academic stars a "hunting license" to work on broad areas: Victor Fuchs on economics of health care, David Mechanic on the organization of medical care, Eli Ginzberg on the health care workforce, and William Schwartz on the costs of health care. In many ways, these scholars helped build a social science understanding of health care beyond the previous work done on hospitals.

The early efforts in training social scientists, especially economists and sociologists, were fruitful. Nevertheless, they were limited in terms of the number of scholars trained and disciplines involved. The Foundation's commitment to these training efforts was very short. Also, the demand for such training, at least among economists, was low.

By 1992, with the authorization of the Scholars in Health Policy Research and the Investigator Awards in Health Policy Research programs, the Foundation had instituted a more strategic way of developing the health policy research capacity of the social science workforce. Authorization of these programs also demonstrated a longer-term commitment by the Foundation to these efforts.

Under these programs, the Foundation was able to permit more freedom than it allowed in traditional research grantmaking. Most Foundation research grantmaking (with the exception of the great men awards) was directed toward research in specified topic areas, such as on health care costs. Those winning Investigator Awards and those selected as Scholars in Health Policy Research were able to pursue health and health care interests beyond what was dictated by the Foundation. For example, although most of the Foundation's efforts still focused on health care problems, many Investigators examined health problems, such as the social determinants of health.

Also, in these programs the Foundation has had to recognize and address the tension between the tight, highly quantified, and focused approach that characterizes research today and the broader, multidisciplinary approach that characterized research up to fifty years ago.

Before the Second World War and in some disciplines since then, scholarship was an individualistic enterprise. Tenure, promotion, and stature depended on individually written articles and books, usually ones about large ideas. Tenure and promotion committees closely scrutinized jointly written articles for the identity of the "true" author. Additionally, those committees frowned upon articles written by a team.

After World War II, and through today, much of the research in medicine, public health, and health services—even in some social sciences—involves large teams of researchers. The research methodology is rigorous, specified, and vetted. It is quantitative, experimental, and quasi-experimental in design. Research results tend to be very narrow and are read by only a small group of researchers.

In the late 1980s, the research portfolio of The Robert Wood Johnson Foundation, as well as the portfolios of other foundations and government agencies, favored tight methodology and narrow topics. The Investigator Awards and the Scholars in Health Policy Research programs attempted to broaden the range of topics, to bring more vision to the field of health policy, and to recruit people with fresh perspectives. In a way, they hearken back to the pre-World War II intellectual tradition, when, at the end of a scholar's career or after his or her death, colleagues and former students produced a *Festschrift,* an edited book celebrating the accomplishments of the individual scholar. The issue of the *Journal of Health Politics, Policy and Law* on Kenneth Arrow is a modern *Festschrift.*

When these programs are successful, they create public intellectuals whose works are read by a broad audience and whose influence extends beyond a narrow academic readership limited to one field (or in some cases even to a subfield). Nevertheless, both types of researcher are important to accomplishing the mission of the Foundation.

Notes

1. Davidson, S., and colleagues. "Evaluation of the Program for Faculty Fellowships in Health Care Finance." (unpublished) The Robert Wood Johnson Foundation, 1991. An updated report on the program appears on the Foundation's Website (www.rwjf.org).
2. Palmer, J., and colleagues. "Evaluation Report to The Robert Wood Johnson Foundation on the Scholars in Health Policy Research Program." (Unpublished) The Robert Wood Johnson Foundation, 2001.
3. Lewin Group. "Investigator Awards in Health Policy Research: Program Assessment. (Unpublished) The Robert Wood Johnson Foundation, 2000.
4. Arrow, K. "Uncertainty and the Welfare Economics of Medical Care." *American Economic Review,* 1963, *53,* 941–973.
5. *Journal of Health Politics, Policy and Law,* 2001, *26*(5).

9

The Robert Wood Johnson Community Health Leadership Program

Paul Mantell

Editors' Introduction

A large philanthropy working at the national level can easily gravitate toward supporting well-established organizations and professionals with impressive credentials. It is crucial, however, to understand that improvements in health and health care come not only from established actors working at the national and state levels but also from people and organizations striving to improve conditions at the community level.

The Foundation's stature may be based largely on its national policy and program activities, but it devotes a significant amount of its resources to supporting local activities. The Local Initiative Funding Partners program, for example, supports efforts devised and carried out by local foundations.[1] Faith in Action, now one of the Foundation's signature programs, supports local interfaith coalitions whose members provide volunteer caregiving to people with chronic health conditions.[2]

The Robert Wood Johnson Community Health Leadership Program is another such program. It identifies local leaders working to improve health or health care, celebrates their contribution, and gives their effort a boost with a modest amount of financial support and the imprimatur of the Foundation's name. It is one of the staff's favorite programs because of the immediacy of the leaders' contributions. Many Foundation programs involve bank shots in their effort to bring improvements to society; this one gives a sense of a direct hit.

This chapter was written by award-winning author Paul Mantell, who is working on a series of brief biographies of all ninety-one winners of The Robert Wood Johnson Community Health Leadership Award. In it, Mantell examines the subtle role of the program, which starts by honoring successful individuals and then capitalizes on the visibility that a Foundation award can bring to further energize them and expand their influence. The program also demonstrates the roles that convening, networking, technical assistance, and seed money can play in helping individuals make a difference in their community.

1. See Wielawski, I. M. "The Local Initiative Funding Partners Program." In *To Improve Health and Health Care 2000: The Robert Wood Johnson Foundation Anthology.* San Francisco: Jossey-Bass, 2000.

2. See Jellinek, P., Gibbs Appel, T., and Keenan, T. "Faith in Action." In *To Improve Health and Health Care 1998–1999: The Robert Wood Johnson Foundation Anthology.* San Francisco: Jossey-Bass, 1998. See also the report on this program on the Foundation's Website (www.rwjf.org).

—w— **E**very year since 1993, The Robert Wood Johnson Community Health Leadership Program has honored ten outstanding but largely unrecognized leaders in the field of community health who have created or significantly improved health services within their community. Many of them have fought through personal hardship, and all have made sacrifices to improve the health of their communities. Here are three of their stories.

Ron Brown

When Ron Brown was seven years old, he was at home with six of his brothers and sisters when their mother's clothing caught fire as she tried to light a kerosene stove. Horrified and helpless, he watched as she burned to death. Subsequently, Brown blamed himself for not being able to save her. This early trauma, and the guilt that resulted from it, led him into drug abuse, and ultimately to prison.

For many people, that would have been the end of the road, but Ron Brown was determined to turn his life around. He resolved to devote himself to helping those people—especially women and children—who were homeless, incarcerated, or otherwise disabled by their addiction to drugs.

In 1977, at the age of twenty-two, Brown was released from prison and found his way to Detroit's Rubicon-Odyssey House. After graduating from the Rubicon recovery program, he became an Odyssey House employee, and by 1987 he was the head of Rubicon's satellite program in Flint, Michigan—a city that, like Detroit, had fallen on hard times.

That same year, Rubicon was forced to close its doors on short notice, and its clients were put at risk. Brown's satellite clinic was still functioning, however, and with $200, some food stamps, and fierce determination, Brown told Rubicon's clients in Detroit that anyone who wanted to follow him to Flint (about seventy miles northwest) would be welcome. They would be treated, and would not be turned away, no matter what.

Several of those people took him at his word, and so did a therapist nurse and two senior residents. This skeleton crew struggled desperately to keep the now-overtaxed Flint Odyssey House afloat. "We had to get some more money," Brown recalls. "We just hustled. We washed cars. We collected donations. We salvaged food from the previous program. They had freezers with liver, and we ate liver for several weeks, breakfast, lunch, dinner. We just toughed it out, getting donations every day for our daily operational basic needs."

Five years later, under Brown's leadership, Flint Odyssey House had grown from one building that offered treatment for fifteen people to a campus with forty buildings providing a variety of programs:

- A long-term residency drug treatment center for the indigent
- A transitional housing program for homeless former substance abusers
- An AIDS outreach project providing prevention services to street drug users
- A Health Awareness Center linking people in the neighborhood with health care services
- Freedom Schools, offering community children teachings in life skills such as grammar, manners, etiquette, organization, self-esteem, and leadership
- Day care for children of residents, enabling parents to attend school or work—an Odyssey House requirement
- Community coalitions and block clubs that paint houses, fences, and garages; clean vacant lots and sidewalks; and renovate and repair the homes of community residents, most of them senior citizens
- The Treat the Streets Program, turning former crack houses into viable low-income housing, built and renovated by the men and women in the residential program. When the patients finish treatment, they're allowed to live in the homes they've renovated. This approach gives homeless people a place to call

their own, gives indigent recovering addicts job skills and self-esteem, and helps rehabilitate the neighborhood.

In 1996, Ronald Brown was honored for his achievements with The Robert Wood Johnson Community Health Leadership Award.

Emma Torres

In 1969, when Emma Torres was thirteen years old, her parents took her out of school and emigrated from Mexico to the United States. In California, she worked in the fields along with her parents, aunts, uncles, and cousins—one of the thousands of migrant workers, many underage, who harvest the foods for Americans' tables. Housing for such workers is often substandard, their working conditions are frequently unhealthy and unsafe, and their access to health care and other services is impeded by an array of barriers.

When Cesar Chavez and his farm workers' union organizers came to the Salinas Valley, Emma and her family were working there, and they became strong supporters of the movement, helping to feed the crowds of workers who flocked to Chavez's banner. They were beaten one day in an ambush in San Lucas, California, while police stood by and even helped. By the age of sixteen, Emma Torres had been targeted as one of the movement's leaders—and thrown in jail. But the farm workers' union had won a part of its battle with the growers. Over time, small improvements continued, though the farm workers' overall plight has continued to be severe.

At age nineteen, Emma Torres married a fellow farm worker, with whom she dreamed of starting a family. By the age of twenty-three, she had one child, and another on the way. That year, her young husband was found to have leukemia. He died at twenty-six, leaving her with two young children and dim prospects for the future.

Throughout her husband's illness, Torres had to travel a long distance to and from the hospital where he was being treated. With almost no command of English, she found it difficult communicating their needs to service providers. "We had always worked," she recalls. "We had never depended on any service or anything. It was very bad for me to go through the services." She became determined to change these conditions.

Torres knew that education was important to her future, so in 1979, after enlisting her mother to help with child care, she enrolled in a trade school, taking English classes and getting a GED. To improve her typing skills to make herself eligible for a job at the local Women, Infants, and Children, or WIC, center, Torres rose before dawn and arrived at school in time to practice. The trip was a long one, because she shared a house with her mother across the border in Mexico.

This was a difficult period, a time of self-doubt and despair. Neighbors and family members called her selfish for leaving her mother to raise her children. Her self-esteem was low. "They said, 'You're a widow, you should be weeping at home, crying your heart out, and letting everybody else feel sorry for you and take care of you,'" she recalls. "But anger gives me strength to do things. I told my mother, 'Do you think they will feed me if I stay home? I have something in mind I want to do, and I don't care about anything else.'"

She got the job at WIC.

Later, Torres worked for a year as a consultant on a pilot perinatal project called Healthy Start. Her assignment for 1988 was to recruit people from the community to serve as lay health workers. Like her, they had to be representative of their community economically, socially, educationally, and linguistically. The idea was that these workers, once trained, would fill a gap in the health care system by tending to the health needs of migrant farm worker women.

In 1989, Torres went on to serve as a migrant liaison for a local community health center, the Valley Health Center Clinic in Somerton, Arizona. Here she developed the Western Migrant Network Tracking System, coordinating and assisting with medical services as workers migrated in and out of state. The program, like most of her creations before and since, operated on an extremely limited budget. Torres often wound up driving clients a considerable distance to medical appointments. She also translated educational materials, coordinated outreach activities, and conducted bilingual nutrition education classes—all in addition to her regular duties at the center.

In 1991, Torres was recruited to open new community lay health worker programs in western Arizona, using the same principles as Healthy Start, but expanding into new areas such as substance abuse and pesticide awareness. The new organization, *Promotores Campesinos* (Health Promotion for Field Workers), provoked fierce resistance in the medical community. Torres had to convince many doctors that well-trained lay health care workers were not a threat to public health, but an asset. Her efforts succeeded, and the programs took root. Today, *Promotores Campesinos* is considered a model for community lay health worker programs around the nation.

Her next venture was another pilot project: a mobile unit bringing health care to migrants in the fields where they worked. Inaugurated in 1994, the MOMOBIL quickly became a successful model project, and Emma Torres began to loom large in Arizona-Mexico border area health care circles. In 1997, she became project manager of *Puentes de Amistad* (Bridges of Friendship), a substance abuse prevention partnership in Yuma, Arizona. There she took on responsibility for developing a staff, finding volunteers, creating coalitions, and conducting community outreach.

Her program *Campesinos sin Fronteras* (Farm Workers Without Borders) coordinates programs on both sides of the border with Mexico, serving workers who frequently cross back and forth.

In 1999, Emma Torres was honored with the Community Health Leadership Award.

Ly-Sieng Ngo

Cambodia's Khmer Rouge unleashed their greatest fury on the country's educated classes, but a young woman named Ly-Sieng Ngo managed to survive the killing fields and was one of the few upper-class, educated Cambodians among the thousands of refugees arriving in Seattle. She could read, write, and speak French, and even a little English. She quickly landed a job as an interpreter at a Seattle health center.

There she witnessed the great pain and profound needs of the Cambodian refugee community, and she began to find ways to help. If people had no food, she found some for them, or showed them how to take the bus to the food bank. If they were unable to take the bus, she did their errands for them. If their child was sick, she would visit and help the family decide whether to go to the emergency room. She attended pregnant women when they went into labor, interpreting for them with the hospital staff.

But Ngo couldn't shake her own awful memories. They haunted her every night, and conventional therapy wasn't helping. Then one weekend, on a solo trip to a friend's cabin in the woods, Ngo found that, for some reason, quilting seemed to make her feel better. If it worked for her, she wondered, why not for others?

When she returned to Seattle, she founded a women's sewing circle, and the results were dramatic. The women began opening up—sharing stories, food, and friendship. They were healing each other's psychological wounds and reawakening one another's interest in life. They were using health facilities much less often. Some no longer required antidepression medication.

When a small retail space in the local hospital fell vacant, Ngo saw an opportunity. "Everything just happened at the right time," she recalls. "The store was available with very little rent, and my women had enough quilts to sell. And then we were on the front page of the *Seattle Times*! And we sold our quilts like hot cookies! It was a miracle."

Ngo was moving ahead on other fronts as well. She trained and evaluated new interpreters. She organized a volunteer network to help people in need of preventive health care. She developed and conducted AIDS education workshops for Cambodian men and their wives. She visited China to study herbal medicine, with the express purpose of providing extra care to personal friends who were sick with AIDS.

Ngo's combination of caring and expertise has allowed her to promote appropriate Western health care practices among Asian patients without undermining their own health beliefs or cultural practices. In 1985, she became a certified community health advocate. She addressed conferences and meetings of American medical providers, speaking about Cambodian culture and appropriate use of interpreters. She provided individual and family health education activities in nutrition, family planning, and prenatal care. Ly-Sieng Ngo has helped sensitize two communities—providers and patients—to cultural differences, and to build an atmosphere of trust between them.

For her achievements, she was honored in 1994 with the Community Health Leadership Award.

—ɯ— The Beginning of the Program

The idea for the Community Health Leadership Program came out of conversations in 1991 among program staff members at The Robert Wood Johnson Foundation who felt that more needed to be done to recognize the leaders behind local initiatives—people who might not be eminent or nationally known but were nevertheless effective, innovative, and courageous leaders in community health. Terrance Keenan, then a Foundation vice president and currently a special consultant to the Foundation, was one of those involved in the program's conception. He recalls, "From our earlier efforts in community health, particularly in support of setting up school-based clinics, we found that persevering, outstanding, committed individuals could do something about getting a community-based health service project under way, often amid great controversy and against great odds."

The Robert Wood Johnson Foundation's staff members hoped that extending the Foundation's recognition to such community health leaders would help legitimize and elevate their work. As expressed in the proposal for the program, the aim of the Community Health Leadership Program was "to provide recognition, through financial awards and technical assistance, for the contributions grassroots community health leaders make to achieving The Robert Wood Johnson Foundation's mission and goals, and to enhance the capacity of these individuals to have more permanent and widespread impact on our nation's health care problems."

Catherine Dunham, a newly arrived special adviser to Steven Schroeder, the Foundation's president, was, according to Keenan, "instrumental in stressing the importance of the fact that these individuals, many of whom did not come with high academic credentials, could nevertheless be catalysts for change on serious, important issues." Dunham, who was hired for her expertise in state government but has a background in community health as well, was asked to head the National Program Office, or NPO, and has served in that position ever since. Third Sector New England, an innovative resource center for nonprofit organizations in Boston, serves as the program's National Program Office. (Dunham is national program director for Third Sector as well.) "Above all, it's the inspiration factor that makes this program such a joy to work on," Dunham says. "These leaders are amazing people. And what they've accomplished is just incredible."

The Community Health Leadership Program was authorized by the Robert Wood Johnson's board of trustees in 1991, starting with a one-year planning grant. This was followed in 1992 by a three-year implementation grant. With renewals over the program's first nine years, and additional grants to the National Program Office for technical assistance, the Foundation's commitment to this program totaled $14 million through 2000. In 2001, the program was renewed for five years at a level of up to $15 million.

It was clear from the beginning that a successful outreach effort to find grassroots candidates would be crucial to the program's success. After setting up the National Program Office, Dunham and the deputy director, Susan Bumagin, together with Foundation staff, brought together a National Advisory Committee to help structure and set the direction for the program, decide on its nomination and screening procedures, and participate in the selection process. Anna Faith Jones, then president of the Boston Foundation, one of the largest community foundations in the nation, was the committee's first chairperson.

—ᴍ— Direction and Administration

In recognition of the community leaders' achievements, the Foundation awards $120,000 (the amount was raised in 2001 from $100,000) to the organization of their choice (generally their own). The money, which is paid out over a period of up to three years, enables the Community Health Leaders to improve and expand their programs. Up to $15,000 of the award money (formerly $5,000–$7,500) comes in the form of a personal stipend. In addition to the monetary award, the Community Health Leadership Program offers recipients annual retreats, enhanced media coverage, access to legislators, and the opportunity to apply for minigrants for capacity building. The program's renewal in 2001 included an expanded array of options for the leaders.

The National Program Office runs the nomination and selection process, plans the awards ceremony, conducts a needs assessment, and works with awardees on media relations in the region and the local community. It offers technical assistance as well, including advice on how to promote the awardees' work through the media and in the funding community. Training is available in the use of computers, software, and the Internet, as is help with marketing, promotion, networking, and advocacy. Program office staff members also make phone calls and write recommendation letters when a community leader requests it. Dunham encourages the leaders to voice their opinions on policy issues and to get involved in the health care debate as advocates for change.

The National Advisory Committee conducts outreach, initial screening, and review of nominations. Its members include community health leaders as well as others familiar with community health (in recent years, past Community Health Leadership awardees have served on the advisory committee). At the outset of the program, the National Advisory Committee's purview was defined by the goals of The Robert Wood Johnson Foundation; those goals, broadly interpreted, guide its outreach activities and selection criteria. In the mid-1990s, at the urging of awardees, the National Advisory Committee broadened its criteria even further by adopting the World Health Organization definition of health, which embraces physical, emotional, mental, and spiritual aspects. The committee recognized that social and economic stability, along with educational investments, has a direct impact on the health of a community. Domestic violence, environmental pollution, poor housing, and urban violence all come into play under this definition.

As a result of adopting such a holistic definition of health, those receiving awards from the Community Health Leadership Program come from many areas: a superintendent of schools, clergymen, lay workers, administrators, concerned citizens, parents, and others not employed in the more traditional health care arena.

—⬩— The Selection Process

The Community Health Leadership Program seeks out midcareer leaders with five to fifteen years of experience who, as a group, represent a rich diversity of backgrounds, fields, and geographic distribution and have overcome significant challenges to improve access to health care and social services to underserved and isolated people in their communities. These leaders must demonstrate (1) a track record of community-based health services leadership; (2) commitment to a career in community health; (3) commitment to working in underserved areas; and (4) consistency with the Foundation's overall goals.

Nominations for the leadership award can be made by health care consumers, community leaders, health professionals, government officials, or "others who have been personally inspired by people providing essential community health services." The National Advisory Committee seeks nominations through an intensive outreach process that includes use of mailing lists, networking, and hundreds of personal phone calls. Nominators submit a letter of intent, which is screened by NPO staff members. If it is approved, a full nomination packet is sent out roughly six weeks later. The NPO's director and deputy director review all nominations and then hand over the files of the top sixty candidates to the National Advisory Committee, which holds a two-day meeting each year in January to rank the top twenty candidates. NPO staff members then visit the sites to learn more about the work of the nominees and how it connects to the community. After the visits are evaluated and references are checked, the National Advisory Committee selects ten candidates to receive the award. In the program's first year, there were 226 nominations. By 2002, that number had grown to 463. Thus far, 101 people have been chosen as Community Health Leaders (with two winners sharing an award in 1994).

—⟋⟍— The Awards Ceremony

The annual awards celebration for the Community Health Leadership Program has been held every year since 1994 in Washington, D.C. In recent years, the ceremony has taken place at the National Press Club, a facility large enough to accommodate the family and friends of the winners. In spite of the travel time and expense—a significant barrier for some—the hall is always packed. Leading up to the big event, the NPO's communications staff distributes press releases featuring each leader in his or her local media markets. The resulting attention may be brief, but it can make a substantial difference in the awardee's ability to raise more funds, reach a wider audience, and have his or her voice included in health policy forums.

On the days before and after the awards ceremony, NPO staff members, National Advisory Committee members, and past winners meet with the new leaders to familiarize them with the program. In addition, taking advantage of the ceremony's Washington location, the program has teamed up with Project Connect, a Robert Wood Johnson Foundation program that introduces Foundation grantees and awardees to their legislators, to arrange meetings for the new leaders with their representatives and senators. Many of the leaders report improved access to their elected representatives, both national and local. Occasionally the payoff is much larger. Ho'oipo DeCambra of Hawaii, who won a leadership award in 2000, convinced Sen. Daniel Inouye of the need for a new health center.

—⟋⟍— Follow-up

Once the awardees have returned home, staff members of the National Program Office move the process forward, sending the new leaders a budget form and a survey designed to help them organize their thoughts and priorities as to how to use their award money. During the summer and the fall, the NPO's deputy director phones the leaders and, using the completed survey as a guide, conducts a structured interview that gives them an opportunity to refine their ideas about how to use the award money. The leaders next send in proposals and budgets, and after agreement on these has been reached, the NPO disburses the money. There are few restrictions on the use of the money, the main one being that it must be spent within three years. NPO staff members encourage leaders to think long-term, to create as much leverage as they can, and to consider as many options as possible. The Community Health Leadership awardees, not surprisingly, universally praise the flexibility of the program's funding. "It was the first time we ever have had unrestricted funds," one recipient says of the award. "It made us feel a sense of partnership and mutual respect. This kind of funding is funding with dignity."

Using the Award Money to Strengthen Communities

The current award, $120,000, is not a large amount in the context of grantmaking at the national level. But it's important to remember that most community-based operations struggle to raise enough funds just to keep going. Emma Torres's *Puentes de Amistad* had a budget in the $200,000 range the year she won the award, with several projects in need of additional support. Torres was able to shore up these projects and offer a salary to two key volunteers.

"It changed my life entirely," Ly-Sieng Ngo says of her award and the money that came with it. She used it to create a support group for Cambodian men that would provide not just healing but a livelihood as well. Their first project was a furniture manufacturing co-op. But after a short while, the men themselves, most of whom had been farmers in Cambodia, asked Ngo if she could help them set up a landscaping business. She turned to the staff of the NPO for help. "They were very supportive and well-organized," she says. "They had expertise in setting up a business and could connect us with people who could help us." The business is now booming, bringing the men increased self-esteem as they take pride in supporting their families and feel secure in their financial future.

Ron Brown's initial plan was to use the funds from the award to create an annuity plan for Odyssey House's long-serving staff. But when he discovered that an old-age home in the neighborhood was about to close its doors, he could not turn away from the need to keep the residents in their home. He used the money to buy the property, saving it and keeping it open to this day.

Supplementary Minigrants and Workshops

In 1996, the Community Health Leadership Program began offering technical assistance in areas beyond spending the award money. The first such assistance was in the form of a workshop for leaders in using the Internet. In 1998, The Robert Wood Johnson Foundation began providing additional support for such capacity-building workshops.

In addition, the NPO has used its technical assistance budget to make minigrants of $3,000-$5,000 to individual leaders. According to national program director Catherine Dunham, these minigrants have been one of the most important features of the entire program (minigrants were made a formal part of the program in the 2002 reauthorization). "I sometimes feel we get even more bang for the buck out of those tiny but precisely targeted grants than we do out of the award funds themselves," she says.

A good example is a 2001 minigrant given to Harry Weinstock, the director of the Brain Injury Association of Virginia and a recipient of a Community Health Leadership Award in 1997. The $4,000 grant was to help develop a strategy to educate legislators about brain injury. When the March legislative session ended, every program in Virginia was cut—except for brain injury programs. When Weinstock spoke to legislators afterward, they told him that the education his group had given them had made a crucial difference. The consultant hired to conduct the training was recently named commissioner of the Department of Rehabilitative Services, the state agency designated to serve people with brain injury. He invited Weinstock to serve on a work group that will help shape that agency's future. All from a $4,000 minigrant!

The Annual Retreat

The NPO arranges an annual retreat for award recipients that takes place in a different city every year. These gatherings, also attended by program staff members, guest speakers, and workshop leaders, amount to a network and support group.

They include a site visit to a local leader's organization. The 2001 retreat, in Memphis, featured the Rev. Kenneth Robinson's St. Andrew AME Church and its many programs for Memphis residents. The church runs programs focusing on the health of the mind, body, and spirit. It has also been buying up derelict properties and renovating the spaces for affordable housing. Retreat participants toured Robinson's programs, as well as the new Hope and Healing Center for healthy living and disease prevention, funded by local faith-based organizations. (Robinson, a 1999 Community Health Leadership Program Award winner, is chairman of the board of the Hope and Healing Center.)

Most Community Health Leadership Program awardees greatly value the program's annual retreats. Just getting together with others who are engaged in similar work and struggles is healing and energizing for the Leaders. "Each time I come back from the retreats, it boosts me up to another level of recovery," Ly-Sieng Ngo says. For Ngo, who still suffers occasional posttraumatic stress, that is no small statement.

According to Emma Torres, "It's like they're part of a great big family I belong to. Whenever I think, 'This is too much, this is too hard, I don't want to do this anymore,' I remember them, and the struggles they have been through. And if I gave them a call, I know they would immediately try to help me."

Benefiting from the Enhanced Credibility of the Community Leaders

Perhaps the greatest effect of receiving the Community Health Leadership Award is the credibility it confers on its recipients. Getting such an endorsement from the largest foundation in the field of health and health care can be transforming for a new or struggling nonprofit organization. It can have a continuing effect, especially in the area of fundraising.

Emma Torres reports that she is now regarded as an authority on migrant worker health issues and is widely sought after for her leadership. She serves on the board of several organizations dealing with such issues as tobacco use, HIV, perinatal health, and cultural competence. In 2000, she became the first Hispanic to run for city council in her home town of Yuma, Arizona, which has a population that is mostly Hispanic. Running on short notice, she fell just short but is considering running again after she has completed her college education.

Another benefit of the award is the media attention that comes with it. Although seizing the national media spotlight has been an uphill struggle, the extensive local media play that leaders typically receive has often had a tremendous return. When Ly-Sieng Ngo returned to Seattle, she found herself the object of intense media attention. "Reporters came to the clinic to interview me, and they put me on the front page the next day," she says. "After that, people kept calling to find out about what I do, ask for advice, ask about my experiences—and it continues."

—ᴍ— Lessons About Leadership

Leadership has to be nurtured, and such nurturing requires knowledge of the components of successful leadership. The attempt to define the essence of leadership is also in the interest of the leaders themselves. Having shouldered responsibilities within their organization, they now need to identify and groom new leaders to take over when they move on. What is it that has made Ron Brown such an effective leader despite his lack of training for such a role? In his own words, "I don't think you can train people like there's a program." Nevertheless, there are some common, identifiable threads that seem to define leadership, at least in the arena of community health.

An article by Constance Pechura, a senior program officer at The Robert Wood Johnson Foundation, and Peter Lee, a Community Health Leadership Award recipient in 1995, described the program and briefly profiled some of the awardees.[1] The authors' view of the essentials of leadership was, in part:

> **Be Quiet and Listen**   Too often health professionals and groups decide what the problems are in a given community without street-level confirmation. Although health workers are well-intentioned, they often go into communities and dictate exactly what help and assistance will be given. They are also often surprised that the communities do not take advantage of the "wonderful" programs they have established. Even when surveys are done to elicit input from individuals and groups from the community, they can be biased by the prejudgments of the investigators. For example, by asking about certain problems (teenage pregnancy, drugs, or access to health care), the investigators may miss the most pressing needs of a community (isolated

elders, infant mortality, lead poisoning). Getting information from community individuals and groups before establishing an intervention may be difficult, but it is a critical step in serving that community.

See Beyond the Obvious   Many health leaders have a vision that is larger than medical care and incorporates a sense of the complex relationships among physical, social, economic, and other aspects of life in a community. Health work focused too narrowly on one specific problem or a specific intervention can miss important opportunities for change.

Network to Build Bridges   Networking essentially involves building bridges to varied community subgroups and persuading people from communities, agencies, and programs to contribute collectively to the solutions for community issues. Many of the Community Health Leadership Program awardees found that they needed to build bridges across language, institutional, and other barriers. They were able to bring a variety of stakeholders to the table and to help them see their relations to one another and to their communities.

Take Care of Yourself   Most community health leaders forget that self-care is a valuable skill that protects and strengthens their programs and vision. Some Community Health Leadership Program Award recipients have found effective methods to reduce stress; others have been helped to recover from their own trauma by their community health work, and still others have used their experiences in survival and self-care to inspire their community health work.

In 1997, The Robert Wood Johnson Foundation commissioned a monograph on leadership, using the stories of twelve program leaders as its major focus. Richard Couto and Stephanie C. Eken wrote the monograph, which was published in 2002.[2] The authors concluded that leadership entails compassion, inspiration and support for others to change individually, inspiration for people to work together, and delegation of the glory attached to success. The authors also stressed commitment to the details of change efforts, as well as to the long haul of change. They identified the common tasks of leadership as coping with constant change, with inherent conflict, and with the need to collaborate. In looking at the Community Health Leadership Program Award recipients, the authors found that community—the willingness to take responsibility for one another—constitutes the firmest common foundation for leadership.

—ɯ— Evaluating the Program

The Alpha Center for Health Planning—now the Center for Health Policy Research—evaluated the Community Health Leadership Program in 1997. The assessment consisted of a written questionnaire sent to forty-nine awardees (thirty-two questionnaires were returned); a telephone survey of twenty-eight awardees, nominators, and community leaders; and site visits to five of the awardees' programs. According to all concerned, the evaluation was conducted under severe time constraints, making it difficult for the investigator to make recommendations that were anything more than tentative. Here are key findings and recommendations of the evaluation:

- Awardees maintained significant dedication to their work and organization despite new career opportunities resulting from the award.

- The support from the National Program Office was greatly appreciated; exploration as to how to maximize support from that office should be considered.

- The methodology and the approaches used to publicize the program and stimulate nominations should be enhanced to identify leaders in needy communities.

- Developing creative approaches to the annual meeting could produce higher benefits.

- Technical assistance on public relations and obtaining additional funds as a result of the award would extend the economic and programmatic impact.

- More active contact with former awardees would promote greater interest in the Foundation's goals.

- Greater specificity, during the post-award period, about the award program conditions for receipt and use of funds would minimize disappointment.

- The process for identifying nominees and selecting recipients should be reviewed.

In response to the evaluation, the National Program Office reviewed and revised its written materials. However, NPO staff members disagreed with some of the evaluation's more critical findings. They pointed out flaws in the study methodology, the rushed nature of the evaluation, and the natural limitations posed by funding constraints and the small number of participants. The evaluator agreed that perhaps some findings might have been distorted by the time limitations placed on the evaluation.

The awardees themselves, interviewed by phone over the past two years, report improved relationships and goodwill in the community, increased community recognition, increased opportunity for regional and national involvement in community health issues and health care reform, enhanced personal honor and sense of meaning, increased leverage for other funding sources, and (most important) increased credibility for themselves and their projects overall.

—〰— Enhancing the Program

In October 2001, the Community Health Leadership Program was reauthorized for $15 million over a five-year period, and the goals were expanded from simply honoring and celebrating grassroots leaders to "enhancing their capacity to address difficult health care problems of their communities." This function had become more and more prominent within the program as the years progressed. Robert Wood Johnson Foundation program staff members have also recognized the potential to develop the Community Health Leadership Program leaders as a resource network for the Foundation.

Under the renewal, the amount of the award was increased to $120,000 per recipient, including $105,000 to the recipient's institution and $15,000 to the recipient to cover professional development and travel. In addition, program "enhancements" were funded: (1) $2.1 million for organizational capacity-building and leadership development activities (peer assistance and mentoring, a leadership institute, assessment tool development, organizational development grants, and a sabbatical program); and (2) $750,000 for research and documentation of leaders' approaches and lessons learned, and development of policy briefs to disseminate lessons learned.

The enhancements are expected to increase the impact of the award for each recipient's institution, and to result in sharing lessons with policy makers, government agencies, community health agencies, and others.

—ᴡᴡ— The Foundation and the Community Health Leaders

National Program Director Catherine Dunham has observed that the Community Health Leadership Program is about more than just recognition. She wants to introduce this growing group of health leaders to the Foundation itself and is quick to point out the contributions the program leaders make to achieving the Foundation's mission and goals. Indeed, some leaders have received grants from the Foundation independent of the Community Health Leadership Program, and in one case a Community Health Program Award recipient, Doriane Miller (1993), was recruited to work as a vice president at the Foundation.

However, The Robert Wood Johnson Foundation has taken only partial advantage of the potential benefits offered by the program, according to Terrance Keenan. "These are not people with long academic CV's with one hundred peer-reviewed publications under their names," he says. "They're people who've been in the trenches, who do the work that makes a difference on a day-to-day basis. But they have some very important lessons to teach others about how to create social change."

According to Dunham, as well as members of the Foundation's program and communications staff, lessons from the program's awardees could be applied to more of the Foundation's national programs. The Foundation has commissioned profiles of Community Health Leadership Program Award recipients that are accessible on the Foundation's Website (www.rwjf.org). These profiles could help make Foundation program staff members more aware of the leaders' work, so that when a spot on a national advisory committee or program that deals with community-based health issues comes up, this ready-made pool of grassroots community health leaders would be considered.

—⚏— **Conclusion**

In summing up the Community Health Leadership Program's efforts, Terrence Keenan says, "I personally regard it as being in the best tradition of philanthropy: identifying outstanding leaders who otherwise wouldn't get recognition, acknowledging them, and helping support their work. It recognizes how things get done at the really local community level—it recognizes that kind of initiative, that perseverance, that special vision that characterizes this group of leaders." Or, as Tom Chapman, who conducted the program's outside assessment, put it, "Programs like the Community Health Leadership Program are at the heart of what the Foundation should be all about."

Notes

1. Pechura, C. M., and Lee, P. "Beyond Theory: Lessons from Community Health Leaders." *CORO Leadership Review,* June 2000, pp. 66–67.
2. Couto, R., and Eken, S. *To Give Their Gifts: Health, Community, and Democracy.* Nashville, Tenn.: Vanderbilt University, 2002.

Communications

10

The Covering Kids Communications Campaign

Susan B. Garland

Editors' Introduction

The Robert Wood Johnson Foundation has integrated its communications work with its program activities to a degree unusual in philanthropy. Through a series of chapters in the *Anthology*, we have tried to capture the nature and the scope of communications within the Foundation.[1] In this chapter, Susan B. Garland, who was an award-winning correspondent for *Business Week* and is now a freelance writer, examines a major Foundation-funded communications campaign that supported its Covering Kids® program.

In 1997, Congress passed the State Children's Health Initiative Program, or SCHIP, and allocated to the states a total of $48 billion over ten years to expand health insurance coverage for children in poor and near-poor families. To help ensure that the programs would be implemented effectively in all fifty states, the Foundation made one of its largest sets of investment ever. Through the Covering Kids program, a total of $47 million has been allocated to coalitions in all fifty states to help them enroll children in the SCHIP and Medicaid programs.[2] In 2000, the Foundation authorized an additional $26 million for an ambitious communications campaign to publicize the availability of health insurance for children.

In this chapter, Garland analyzes the strategy and the approaches used in the communications campaign. The goal of the campaign was to get potentially eligible families to call a phone number for information about how to enroll in their state's children's health insurance program. To do this, the Foundation obtained the services of a major advertising agency and a prestigious market research firm. Working with the National Program Office for the Covering Kids program, they developed a series of ad campaigns that ran in selected markets throughout the country.

Although the number of callers to the hotline increased immediately after the ad campaigns, there remain some unanswered questions. Among them, the most important are whether callers to a hotline took the next step and enrolled their children in the program, and whether massive communications campaigns such as this are cost-effective. There is little solid evidence to answer either question.

Despite these open questions, the story of the Covering Kids communications campaign is an important one for other philanthropies or organizations considering a similar campaign to get people to take action to help themselves.

---

1. Frank Karel provided a retrospective look in "'Getting the Word Out': A Foundation Memoir and Personal Journey." In *To Improve Health and Health Care 2001: The Robert Wood Johnson Foundation Anthology.* San Francisco: Jossey-Bass, 2001; Victoria D. Weisfeld focused on the Foundation's radio and television work in "The Foundation's Radio and Television Grants, 1987–1997." In *To Improve Health and Health Care 1998–1999: The Robert Wood Johnson Foundation Anthology.* San Francisco: Jossey-Bass, 1998; Marc S. Kaplan and Mark A. Goldberg examined a media campaign connected with the Foundation's Health Tracking program in "The Media and Change in Health Systems." In *To Improve Health and Health Care 1997: The Robert Wood Johnson Foundation Anthology.* San Francisco: Jossey-Bass, 1997; Digby Diehl discussed the Foundation's support of community radio in "Sound Partners for Community Health." In *To Improve Health and Health Care 2001: The Robert Wood Johnson Foundation Anthology.* San Francisco: Jossey-Bass, 2001.

2. The Foundation's efforts to make health insurance available for children is examined in Holloway, M. Y. "Expanding Health Insurance for Children." In *To Improve Health and Health Care 2000: The Robert Wood Johnson Foundation Anthology.* San Francisco: Jossey-Bass, 2000.

—ɯ— Every day, millions of American families face the twin threats of medical disaster and financial devastation. Because health care costs so much, many children who are not covered by insurance don't receive even routine care, from dental checkups to immunizations. According to a survey sponsored by The Robert Wood Johnson Foundation, one in five parents of uninsured children was forced to skip needed medical treatment for a sick child because they didn't know how they would pay for it.[1] If a child is hospitalized, parents can face catastrophic bills.

Regrettably, many families don't realize that they may be eligible for government-sponsored health coverage for their children. Medicaid is the largest publicly financed program of health services for children. It provides free coverage to low-income kids. In August 1997, Congress expanded coverage with the passage of the State Children's Health Insurance Program. SCHIP enables families whose income exceeds the Medicaid limit to sign up their children for health insurance. The states administer the SCHIP program and have some leeway in setting eligibility standards. In about one-third of the states, parents who earn 200 percent of the poverty level (the federal poverty level in 2002 was $18,100 for a family of four) can enroll their children for free or low-cost coverage; some states exceed these income levels and others fall below them. Under both Medicaid and SCHIP, the state governments share the costs with Washington.

Health reformers hailed SCHIP as a godsend for the many working families that couldn't afford private coverage but earned too much to qualify for Medicaid. These parents either don't get family insurance coverage at their jobs or can't afford their share of the monthly premiums. Still, despite the existence of generous government coverage programs, 8.5 million children—11.6 percent of all kids—were not covered by health insurance in 2000, according to the U.S. Census Bureau.[2] Most of them live in a family where at least one parent is working. Even more troubling, more than half of these uninsured children were eligible for SCHIP or Medicaid but had not signed up for coverage.

—ᴍ— Background to the Communications Campaign: The Covering Kids Initiative

For years before Congress passed SCHIP, The Robert Wood Johnson Foundation had been concerned about lackluster enrollment among Medicaid-eligible children. Since the failure of President Clinton's health reform plan in 1994, the Foundation had been seeking ways to increase enrollment of eligible children who were not participating in Medicaid. Foundation staff members reasoned that community leaders should go into the neighborhoods, find eligible youngsters, and sign them up. In July 1997, the Foundation approved a new program to do just that. Covering Kids: A National Health Access Initiative for Low-Income, Uninsured Children authorized $13 million for community-based coalitions of health care advocates and government officials in fifteen states and local communities. The Foundation chose the Southern Institute on Children and Families, a public policy organization based in Columbia, South Carolina, as the National Program Office. Sarah C. Shuptrine, the institute's president, was named to head the program office.

Only a month after Covering Kids was approved, Congress passed SCHIP. Recognizing the potential of Covering Kids to help many more youngsters than first envisioned, in July 1998 the Foundation expanded the program to cover the entire country. The expansion added another $34 million to create coalitions in all fifty states, 170 communities, and the District of Columbia. The program was to cover a three-year period, from 1998 to 2001. (In April 2001, the Foundation, building on Covering Kids, approved a four-year, $68 million initiative called Covering Kids and Families.)

Covering Kids sought to attack the enrollment problem from three angles. First, the coalitions that the states and localities created would reach out and enroll eligible children at schools and other community-based organizations. Second, the coalitions would tackle the complex application process to make it easier for an eligible family to sign up. To this end, the coalitions would help the states remove burdensome and unnecessary questions and tasks (such as a face-to-face interview) not required for determining eligibility, thus significantly shortening the application form and process. Third, the initiative would prod states to coordinate SCHIP and Medicaid. In many states, the two programs had separate offices, applications, and requirements; without coordination, a child rejected by one program was not automatically considered for the other.

—ᴡ— The Communications Campaign

Even as the coalitions' activities grew, The Robert Wood Johnson Foundation remained concerned that the federal government was not actively publicizing SCHIP and Medicaid, and that the states had not touched millions of available federal dollars targeted for children's health care. Foundation staff members were convinced that a nationally coordinated advertising effort, coupled with grass-roots and outreach activities that generated information and messages backed by high-level market research, would work. If the right message were created, they believed, low-income parents could be persuaded to take the first step: calling the hotline. In January 2000, the Foundation decided to "raise the ante," as Stuart Schear, a senior communications officer at the Foundation who spearheaded the effort, described it. It authorized $26 million for an aggressive communications campaign to increase the visibility of the government programs. In effect, the Foundation was trying to fill a gap left by the federal government.

To run the communications campaign, the Foundation contracted with Greer, Margolis, Mitchell, Burns, & Associates, or GMMB, which creates media campaigns for political candidates and also specializes in public-awareness campaigns, such as the Air Bag and Seat Belt Safety Campaign.

The Covering Kids Communications Campaign had three fundamental strategies. The first was to complement the existing Covering Kids coalitions' outreach effort with a media blitz that would encourage viewers or listeners to call a toll-free government hotline for enrollment assistance (although it was not actively publicizing SCHIP and Medicaid, the Department of Health and Human Services allowed Covering Kids to use its toll-free hotline in its marketing efforts). Four- or five-week media blitzes would be timed to run with high-visibility grassroots enrollment activities organized by the Covering Kids coalitions of health care professionals, business leaders, churches, government officials, schools, and child advocates.

The second strategy was to enlist as partners dozens of national organizations and major corporations, which would encourage their local members and stores to get the word out about government health insurance programs for children. The third strategy was to train local Covering Kids coalition members to develop long-term relations with the press and to deliver research-tested information to their community. The communications professionals would send senior Covering Kids officials to meet with journalists, train local coalition members to reach out to local news organizations, hold press conferences in Washington and in target markets, and advise local outreach workers on how to distribute information to community organizers and eligible families.

In effect, the Covering Kids communications campaign was to operate much like a political campaign, bombarding communities with information from many sources. Annie Burns, a partner in GMMB, described the premise of this saturation strategy: "When parents go to work, they hear a story on the radio, and at night they see the advertising on TV. When they go into a store, they see a poster, and when they go to a back-to-school meeting, the school nurse tells them about Medicaid and SCHIP. When you hit people every place they live their lives, then you increase the likelihood that they will take the step that will bring them closer to getting health insurance for their children."

—⟋⟍— Conducting Market Research

As in most social marketing campaigns, the Covering Kids communications team uses techniques from the world of corporate marketing. But the Foundation's initiative differs from other campaigns in several ways, chief among them its extensive use of in-depth market research to study the motivations of low-income populations.

The Foundation signed on Wirthlin Worldwide, a firm that conducts research and creates advertising messages for General Motors, McDonald's, Boeing, and many other large corporations. Wirthlin was directed to conduct the research and help come up with a set of message concepts that would become the framework for the advertising and for other facets of the communications campaign. "We performed the same level of analysis that we perform for any of our Fortune 100 clients," said Maury Giles, a senior research executive at Wirthlin, who handles the $1 million-plus Covering Kids account.

But marketing cars or hamburgers is different from selling the idea of health coverage to low-income parents. In creating the message framework, Wirthlin knew that a parent's relationship with a child strikes a deep emotional chord, especially for a family where financial survival and responsible parenthood are often competing priorities. With this in mind, the firm recognized that the communications strategy needed to link the tangible benefits of health coverage with the personal values that would motivate these parents to take action.

In the spring of 2000, Wirthlin conducted two-hour, one-on-one interviews in five cities with 114 adults whose children either were enrolled in Medicaid or SCHIP or were likely to be eligible. The interviews targeted four ethnic groups: Caucasian, African American, Latino, and Native American. The firm used a proprietary research methodology that links rational considerations with emotional ones—in this case, the attributes of coverage with the emotions parents have about their role as protector. The insights from the interviews led to the communications framework: all of the ads and materials had to show that being a good parent meant raising successful, healthy children, and enrolling in a program offering low-cost or free health care was a smart choice. This in turn would reduce stress and bring peace of mind.

The conclusion would seem like a given. But the value of the market research, according to Giles, was in eliminating many other possible messages that, on the surface, would seem equally logical. For instance, the researchers had considered a message that would show parents how much healthier their kids would be if they signed up for health coverage. The assumption was that low-income parents didn't see the value of heath care. But, Giles noted, "The parents saw great value in taking their kids to the doctor." They simply couldn't afford it.

The researchers had also been considering a message aimed at overcoming parents' negative feelings about government programs. During June, two focus groups of social service caseworkers told researchers that many families wouldn't sign up because of the social stigma associated with public programs. That's not what low-income families told researchers, though. During the same month, Wirthlin conducted telephone interviews with nearly three thousand parents of eligible children. Seventy-five percent said they believed government health programs based on financial need were "a good thing to help people take care of their families." Only 25 percent said these programs were a "public symbol that I cannot make it on my own." However, they feared that front-office staff at the doctors' offices would treat them rudely.

The biggest obstacle to enrollment, the parents said, was that most of them didn't realize their kids were eligible. Only 22 percent of these parents had ever heard of SCHIP, and most of those aware of the program didn't realize they could qualify. "We went into the market research having listened to the professionals talk about social stigma as being a major barrier to signing up," said Elaine Arkin, a communications consultant retained by the Foundation. "We came out of the research with a different understanding: the biggest barrier was that these families didn't believe they were eligible. Some of these parents work two or three jobs, and they don't assume the government will provide something for them."

—ɯ— The First Ad Campaign: August 2000

By mid-2000, GMMB and Wirthlin were developing the ads. The close relationship between the research and creative teams is unusual in the worlds of both social and corporate marketing. Researchers often leave the scene once they deliver their findings. Agency executives often toss out the research if it slows the flow of their creative juices. But the Foundation would not tolerate such turf battles. It insisted that the creative people work with the research team, and that both of them collaborate with the Covering Kids National Program Office, the grantees, and the national organizations that were carrying out the marketing work.

GMMB produced nine thirty-second television ads for about $450,000, and radio and print ads for $50,000 more. Those production figures did not include the costs of buying air time and newspaper ad space. GMMB wanted high-quality spots that could run alongside product advertising and not turn off prospective "consumers." So it used film instead of videotape and hired professional actors. Persons of all targeted ethnic groups played patients, physicians, and office staff. Because parents in focus groups were concerned about how they would be treated in the waiting rooms, "office personnel" in the spots appeared friendly and cheerful. Some of the ads had a version with Spanish audio and written screen information. The voiceovers for all of the ads could be changed to provide information aimed at audiences in specific states. Public service announcement versions that could run anywhere were also created.

Before airing the advertisements, Wirthlin and GMMB convened four groups of parents of eligible children to view them. Even after viewing the ads many times, the parents didn't realize they were the target audience. The communications team was surprised. "After we mentioned that they could apply, they said, 'No, no, I'm not eligible because I'm working,'" Burns of GMMB recalled. "We told them that from the information they gave us they were eligible. They found it hard to believe." When told they could apply, they started writing down the hotline number. This convinced GMMB and Wirthlin to use an income figure in the voiceovers. In Maryland, for instance, viewers would be told that "even families earning up to $30,000 or more" could get free coverage.

The decision sparked a firestorm. Though Idaho had agreed to become a target market, state officials there worried that the generous income limits would attract too many costly enrollees. Sarah Shuptrine, head of the National Program Office, believed a specific dollar figure would be misleading, since income limits differ by family size. Only a family of four would qualify on the basis of the income figure used in Maryland's ad. A mother with one child would be eligible only if she earned less than $23,000. Shuptrine worried that a mother earning slightly more would feel duped if she applied and was rejected.

Wirthlin convened a second round of focus groups to retest the language. Viewers noted they wouldn't be angry if they were rejected. Shuptrine is still not convinced. "In the focus groups, just using the words 'working families' was very effective," she said.

The four-week wave of coordinated advertising and outreach efforts, known as Back-to-School 2000, started in mid-August in six media markets. The Foundation wanted the ads tested in these six markets before it would decide whether to expand. It also demanded measurable proof of the strategy's effectiveness—in this case, an increase in the number of calls to the hotline. The strategists chose medium-sized markets where advertising costs were reasonable. Targets were also selected on the basis of ethnic and geographical characteristics: Albuquerque, New Mexico, and Fresno, California, for Latinos; Baltimore and

Greenville, North Carolina, for African Americans; and Springfield, Illinois, and Boise, Idaho, for Caucasians. In addition, the strategists chose only those states that were simplifying enrollment procedures. "The last thing we wanted was to go out with a pizzazzy media campaign only to have families turned off by the application process," Shuptrine said.

Though many social marketing campaigns depend on free public service announcements, the Foundation could afford paid advertising. "If you are looking to have a certain impact within a certain time frame with a certain audience, paid advertising gives you more control," GMMB partner Burns said. GMMB bought time during radio and television shows popular with target ethnic groups between the ages of eighteen and thirty-four. The agency made enough buys so parents would see the spots thirty-five times over four weeks. "We weren't just trying to promote awareness, but to actually get people to pick up a phone," said David A. Smith, another GMMB partner. "We wanted to have enough frequency to ensure that our target audience would see it and be motivated to make a call."

The advertising wave coincided with 268 high-visibility Covering Kids enrollment activities in the six target markets as well as in twenty other states. The enrollment activities included health fairs that distributed goody bags with prizes and information; sign-up tables at churches, businesses, festivals, and hospitals; and free immunizations and physicals at community events. To intensify the impact of the ads and the enrollment events, the strategists sought to generate extensive news coverage by releasing some of Wirthlin's research findings. Covering Kids unveiled its communications campaign at press conferences in Washington and in the six markets. The hook that grabbed press attention was the Wirthlin findings that had guided the communications strategy: six out of ten parents of eligible children didn't realize their kids were eligible for government health insurance programs, and 82 percent said they would apply if they knew they would qualify. Covering Kids counted more than fifteen thousand television, radio, and print news stories, which reached about 78.8 million Americans. This included forty TV stories in the target markets, coverage on national networks, and articles in newsmagazines and top newspapers.

From the first, the Foundation sought ways to assess whether the communications strategy was working. News coverage was one measurement. The triple punch of ads, outreach, and news coverage delivered the audience impact the communications strategists sought. Calls to local hotlines in each of the six test markets rose significantly. Because of the extensive national media coverage, calls to the national hotline soared as well, to fifty-eight thousand during August, up from fifteen thousand a month before the campaign. In September, the calls remained high, at thirty-three thousand, which the White House attributed to Covering Kids and its communications campaign. In two control markets—Idaho Falls, Idaho, and Wilmington, North Carolina, where the campaign ran no ads—the number of calls rose very little in comparison. For instance, average weekly calls to the North Carolina hotline from Wilmington rose to 27 during the campaign period, up from a weekly average of 13 calls before the campaign. Meanwhile, calls from Greenville, a target market, rose to 246 during the campaign, up from 33 calls before.

Even during the advertising wave, Wirthlin was evaluating the impact. It interviewed 503 hotline callers in Albuquerque and Greenville to find out what had motivated them to call. Advertising was the main cause; more than 80 percent said they had learned of the telephone number from the ads, and most of the callers said they intended to apply. Fewer than 10 percent of the callers learned from the telephone operators that they were not eligible. Once the advertising wave was over, Wirthlin surveyed three thousand parents in test and comparison markets and found that 58 percent in the test markets had seen the ads, and that one out of four who had seen the ads made a call.

—w— The Second Ad Campaign: March 2001

For the next phase, the strategists returned to the same markets (except for Greenville). Starting in March, during a flu season enrollment drive, the campaign aired the same ads but did not hold press events or release new research. Depending on the market, ads ran five or six weeks. Calls to the national hotline and to hotlines in target markets rose, but the numbers were less than half of what they were the first time around. "It was harder to go back to the same markets and get the coverage again," GMMB's Burns said.

During that phase, Covering Kids expanded to Miami and New Orleans with radio ads only. The campaign wanted to see if radio alone could generate similar results at lower cost. Though hotline calls rose, the increase was not as dramatic as a combined television and radio blitz in the previous phase. Covering Kids had increased its ad spending in this phase, to $1.9 million, but the press coverage reached an audience of only four million. This compared with the $1.8 million spent in the first campaign, which generated national news coverage reaching nearly eighty million Americans.

—⋙— The Third Campaign: August 2001

Seeking a bigger impact in the next phase, the communications team decided to enter new markets for a Back-to-School 2001 campaign. This time, GMMB asked the states to apply to become target markets, expecting that a contest of sorts would attract the most committed grantees. GMMB eventually chose Miami; Tucson; Hartford, Connecticut; Brownsville, Texas; and the District of Columbia.

The Foundation didn't have the resources for an intensive ad campaign nationwide, but the strategists thought they could boost enrollments in nontarget states with a modest national buy. Beyond the money spent in the target markets, the Foundation spent more than $500,000 to buy ad time in thirty-six states on ABC Radio and the Univision Television Network. GMMB believed that such ads in nontarget states could help Covering Kids grassroots organizers generate additional interest in the government health programs. GMMB's Smith recalled, "Organizations conducting news events would have some level of advertising that they could point to. As in the target markets, people would be hearing the messages wherever they went—on the radio and in their doctor's offices."

As it did in Back-to-School 2000, Covering Kids conducted splashy news conferences in Washington and in target markets. Organized by the communications team, the Washington news conference featured Shuptrine, the mayor of the District of Columbia, the New York State health commissioner, the president of the National Association of Chain Drug Stores, and families from several states. Once again, the communications strategists decided that Covering Kids should release new data at the news conferences. Among the statistics that grabbed headlines: one in five parents of uninsured children delayed or skipped medical care for their children because they couldn't pay for it. In part because of the national advertising on Univision and ABC Radio, the news coverage was even bigger this time around, reaching an audience of more than eighty-four million people.

Once again, calls to the national hotline soared, to 47,183 in August, and remained high, at 27,105, in September. Hotline calls in the target markets also rose from precampaign levels in those two months. In Hartford, average weekly calls rose by 166 percent, to 678 during the campaign, up from 255 before. Awareness of the programs rose, too: in 2001, some 54 percent of parents of eligible-but-uninsured children thought their kids were eligible, compared with 36 percent a year earlier.

—ᴡ— Linking Communications with Grassroots Activity

The advertising was not the only factor that led to this increase in calls. The communications team helped the coalitions organize enrollment events for the Back-to-School campaigns. The grassroots activists distributed two million fliers, bookmarks, and other promotional materials with messages backed by market research. Indeed, although the advertising borrows a page from the book on corporate marketing, the grassroots operations have the look and feel of a political campaign, with local and state foot soldiers reinforcing the carefully created communications message.

The communications team works closely on the outreach effort with the National Program Office and the Covering Kids state and local grantees. With guidance from the program office, the states and the communities have developed coalitions among hospitals, social service agencies, schools, and other groups that seek out eligible children and enroll them in government insurance programs. Meanwhile, GMMB has provided extensive technical communications assistance to coalitions, which have had little experience running aggressive marketing and grassroots campaigns.

A case in point: in the Back-to-School 2001 Campaign Action Kit, GMMB offered coalitions a detailed timeline for planning a press conference, with instructions on what they should be doing in the six weeks leading up to the event. The kit included talking points, templates of news advisories and speaker invitations, tips for pitching stories to reporters, and advice on enlisting schools and businesses to get the word out.

The training paid off, with the kind of high-visibility press events that local activists had rarely tried. In Hartford, the Connecticut lieutenant governor kicked off Back-to-School 2001 at a press conference. Also speaking was Guadalupe Arroyo, whose eight-year-old daughter, Connie, suffers from tuberous sclerosis, a genetic condition that causes tumors to grow on the brain. Her husband is an exterminator, and though his employer's health plan covers his two children, out-of-pocket costs for Connie's care are enormous. Arroyo heard about Connecticut's SCHIP program at a PTA meeting, and though she doubted her children would qualify, she applied and was accepted. "When I meet people who don't have insurance, I tell them all about it," Arroyo said several months later.

Besides recruiting Arroyo, the Children's Health Council (the Connecticut grantee) helped organize more than one hundred enrollment and outreach events across the state. Volunteers offered application help at the Bridgeport Zoo. While registering for school, children enrolled in SCHIP. At a Wal-Mart reopening in Manchester, SCHIP organizers inside the store offered raffles. Judith Solomon, executive director of the state-funded council, said that in the past such events at stores and fairs had failed to attract much attention. This time, she said, people were asking questions. She believed the TV ads "legitimized the program," and she has bought a number of ad tapes, which she is pitching to local cable access stations. She also said the technical assistance from GMMB was invaluable. "We never wrote a press release before," she said. "We'll do them from now on."

In addition, GMMB produced fifty-page communications kits for reaching Latino and Native American families. In its Latino kit, the communications team offers advice on recruiting high school students as volunteers, making home visits, setting up enrollment tables at cultural festivals, and working with local businesses. The kit also offers tips on getting the local Immigration and Naturalization Service involved and recruiting *promotoras* (lay health workers).

In Doña Ana County in New Mexico, the Covering Kids pilot has enlisted the INS to encourage immigrants to enroll their U.S.-born children. The pilot there is using *promotoras* to meet with families in their homes. "These are trusted members of the community," says Shelly Almaguer, the Covering Kids program manager in the county. "It's not easy for people on the outside to come in."

—〰— **Partnerships with Nationwide Groups**

A key goal of the communications strategy was to find as many outlets as possible to disseminate information about the government health coverage programs for children. To bolster both its local grassroots operations and the advertising campaign, the communications team recruits national organizations and corporations to help raise the visibility of Medicaid and SCHIP. More than eighty national associations and nonprofits representing educators, faith-based groups, child advocates, unions, and medical professionals are distributing information to their members and the public. They also encourage their local chapters and offices to develop ties to community groups, reinforcing the strength of the local coalitions. The communications team at GMMB designed the promotional materials that these groups distribute.

Linda C. Wolfe, president of the National Association of School Nurses, says the association sends Covering Kids information to eleven thousand members in its newsletter. When a parent visits a school to pick up a sick kid, the nurse can hand over a SCHIP brochure and, in some states, enroll the child on the spot. The American College of Emergency Physicians, which represents fifty-five hundred emergency department directors, has mailed its members Covering Kids posters to hang in the waiting room, brochures to distribute to parents, and advice on running enrollment programs. "Getting more children insured is a high priority for emergency physicians," says Colleen Horn, public relations manager for the college.

Nurses and doctors are natural partners, but large corporations are a harder sell. Still, the Foundation believes that businesses have an important audience for a communications message: a customer base of potential enrollees and part-time employees who are not covered by the company health plan. Kelly Carey, a GMMB vice president, has developed relationships with corporate trade groups and major retailers, mostly pharmacy and grocery chains.

Carey's efforts are paying off. Twenty-five companies in forty-seven states participated in Back-to-School 2001. In March 2002, some twenty-four hundred Albertson's stores in thirty-three states started distributing two hundred million grocery bags emblazoned with the hotline number and sixty-five million advertisements and circulars. CVS is displaying promotional materials in the pharmacy department in two hundred of its stores in Maryland, Virginia, and the District of Columbia. The GMMB strategists customized the materials with the participating company's logo.

For corporations with stores in the local community, participating in Covering Kids enrollment efforts makes good business sense. If more children obtain health coverage, pharmacy departments make more money. Enrollment events bring customers into the store and generate positive publicity. It also has philanthropic appeal. Phillip Schneider, vice president of the National Association of Chain Drug Stores, said it was a "natural mix" for pharmacies and Covering Kids to work together. "Every day pharmacists see mothers come in asking for information about a child's illness," he said. "They don't have the money to fill a prescription."

Carey has also trained social service advocates to approach Main Street businesses and work with the local chains once she's opened doors with corporate headquarters. The advice runs the gamut, from writing letters to company executives to enlisting enough volunteers to operate an enrollment table. One such success: in New Mexico, El Paso Electric agreed to send an informational flyer with its bills.

—⁓— Centralized Control Versus Local Sensitivity

Any initiative that involves so many far-flung players is sure to run into problems. Although the enrollment drives may have appeared to come off without a hitch, the road to getting there was often rocky. The Foundation-GMMB partnership had to balance the need for centrally controlled communications with the preferences of people at the state and local levels. Tensions rose during the months leading up to Back-to-School 2000, since the marketing team had a tight deadline to prepare and test the ads. Those working in the target markets had to approve every word. Each state wanted to use its own brand name for the program, and some wanted to use a local hotline number. A couple of states wanted to mention that the program offered prescription drugs; others wanted to mention that it offered an insurance card. It took dozens of long conference calls to work out the snags.

At times, local sensitivities caught GMMB by surprise. In the March 2001 phase, the communications team believed its Spanish-language TV spots for Univision could run in every Spanish-speaking community across the country—until the Texas grantee told the ad maker that Spanish dialects differed from region to region. So the agency scurried to create several Spanish versions of the same ad to run in different locations.

In some cases, tension arose between the national campaign and some states reluctant to use precious financial resources to pay for health insurance for more children. In other cases, a source of tension was the capacity of states to carry out the program.

—w— The Next Stage

As the communications campaign moved into its final year, the Covering Kids communication team planned a new round of target markets for Back-to-School 2002. Because of the success of the nationwide television and radio ads during the 2001 drive, the Foundation was again placing ads across the country. GMMB was considering "communications boot camps" to train grantees in how to pitch a story to the press, conduct an interview, and stage a press conference.

Foundation staff members believe that coalitions have developed so much expertise in outreach and communications that they can step up enrollment efforts throughout the year; Covering Kids has offered its market research and ad spots to any government agency that wants them. Similarly, they expect that national organizations and corporations will continue many activities without intensive direction from Covering Kids. The campaign will also broaden its outreach to restaurants, video rental companies, and other types of companies that have customers whose kids need health coverage.

Though funding for the communications campaign continues through 2002, grants to states and local pilots under the Covering Kids program began expiring in January 2001. In April of that year, the Foundation approved a new four-year initiative called Covering Kids and Families. The new $55 million program supports coalitions in all fifty states and the District of Columbia working to enroll children eligible for Medicaid and SCHIP and, in up to thirty states, working to enroll eligible adults. Since the communications campaign's funding continues until the end of 2002, the communications team focused its efforts on this new initiative. Wirthlin researched new messages. "We need special strategies to attract adults who are not parents of eligible children," Shuptrine said.

Another focus of the new Covering Kids and Families initiative, as well as of the communications team, was on the issue of "retention." Although Covering Kids attracted new children to Medicaid and SCHIP, many fall off the rolls when their coverage expires. Few states notify families beforehand, and reenrollment can be even more arduous than the initial application process. The communications team developed messages that attempted to keep kids enrolled. Meanwhile, Covering Kids coalitions continued to work with states to simplify the reenrollment process.

—ɯ— Lessons from the Covering Kids' Communications Campaign

Though Covering Kids is unique in many ways, social marketers (especially in the health care field) can look to its communication strategy for lessons in creating their own campaigns.

Awareness gap   The Foundation understood the fallacy of the notion "Build it and they will come." Creating awareness of new services is just as important as building the services themselves. Repetition is important too; an occasional ad or PTA meeting won't have the same impact as a saturation strategy. The Foundation proved that a well-designed campaign could generate enough interest to cause people to pick up the phone. Even so, a significant percentage of eligible parents who saw or heard the ads didn't call to get more information.

Integrated campaign   Foundation officials argue that the advertising and grassroots activities were both important in generating interest among people whose children were potentially eligible for SCHIP or Medicaid. Social marketers considering an integrated approach should think about time-limited campaigns (in this case, four- and five-week blitzes) since, in the case of Covering Kids, this kept enthusiasm high.

Market research   Though it's expensive, market research that pinpoints the most effective message can pay off in the long run, especially if there is strong collaboration between researchers and the media team. When the targets are people with low income, research is particularly important since most ad agencies are unfamiliar with this segment of the population.

Market segmentation   Social marketers must pay close attention to demographics. The Foundation found that although its overall communications framework appealed to all four targeted ethnic groups, subtle differences were taken into account in the final messages. For instance, African Americans connected to the idea of protecting a child, while Latino audiences responded to the financial-stress part of the message. GMMB's having to create several Spanish-dialect versions of the ads underscored the reality that ethnic groups are not homogeneous.

Specifics   Creating an ad heavy in atmospherics does not necessarily prompt a target audience to take a specific action step. The research for the Covering Kids communications campaign showed that parents would place a call because they believed there was a direct benefit to them. That meant the ads had to convey specific information, such as an income eligibility figure or some idea of what the coverage offered (doctor visits, prescription drugs, and so on).

Coalition building   Working with state and local professionals who understand the target population is essential. But building an on-the-ground coalition can be a difficult task, especially if much of the direction is coming from outsiders. Collaboration means open and frank discussion. In Back-to-School 2000, the short period between conception and execution created some tension; a marketing campaign requiring complex partnerships should build in extra planning time.

Wide net   By seeking an array of partners, Covering Kids was able to get out the word in many venues. The participation of churches, advocacy groups, corporations, national organizations, and officials from all levels of government helped ensure that the target audience heard the message repeatedly.

Business outreach   Many advocates of social change are intimidated about approaching businesses. But if a marketer can make an effective pitch, a business can be an ideal partner. It has customers, employees, deep pockets, and its own marketing know-how. Business involvement also can convince a wary target audience that an initiative is worthwhile.

Long-lasting change   Social change doesn't have a time limit, but a marketer's involvement usually does. In this case, the Foundation sought to build a structure that would last long after the Foundation and the communications team departed the scene. Local activists in coalitions have developed close relationships among themselves. The training materials and the market research that Covering Kids has given coalitions deepens their expertise. GMMB also has made public service versions of the ads available to agencies for local marketing efforts.

Removing structural roadblocks   William D. Novelli, a pioneer in social marketing and currently the executive director and chief executive officer of AARP, argued that a campaign's success hinges on whether the target audience can easily make the behavior change the marketer desires. "You don't want them to jump a fence and swim a river to get what they want," he said. In the case of Covering Kids, simplifying the process was essential, from shortening the application form to making sure the hotline worked well. Before Albertson's decided to place the number on grocery bags and in advertising, several vice presidents tested the hotline.

—ᴍᴡ— Conclusion

Although the communications strategists set out to enroll 2.5 million new children in SCHIP and Medicaid, this measurement of success ultimately may be the most difficult to gauge. In 2001, 4.6 million children were enrolled in SCHIP, up from 1.9 million in fiscal year 1999, according to the federal Centers for Medicare & Medicaid Services.[3] But it's difficult if not impossible to tease out the number of enrollments that are due to the Covering Kids communications campaign from enrollment due to other factors. It stands to reason that some of the people who called the toll-free hotline signed up their children for coverage under Medicaid or SCHIP. The communications campaign surveys and data collection all report extensive news coverage, grassroots activities, growth in the number of participants who were spreading the word, a rise in awareness among eligible families, and an increase in hotline calls. This may well mean that many children who otherwise would have remained uninsured are now enrolled and getting medical care when they need it.

Notes

1. Wirthlin Worldwide. "Survey of American Families: Comparison of Households with Insured Children vs. Uninsured Children Eligible for SCHIP/Medicaid Coverage." 2001. (www.coveringkids.org)
2. U.S. Census Bureau. "Health Insurance Coverage: 2000." 2002. (www.census.gov)
3. Centers for Medicare & Medicaid Services. "SCHIP Covers 4.6 Million Children in 2001." 2002. (www.cms.hhs.gov)

A Look Back

11

The Swing-Bed Program

Sharon Begley

Editors' Introduction

Every year, the *Anthology* takes a look back at a program funded by the Foundation some years ago to get a historical perspective on the Foundation's work. This year, the *Anthology* looks back at a program developed in the 1970s, formally called the Rural Hospital Program of Extended-Care Services, to use excess hospital beds in rural areas to deliver long-term care for the frail and disabled. Informally, it was known as "the swing-bed program."

The swing-bed idea arose from a twin set of problems facing rural health care systems: (1) hospitals were built on a scale that often resulted in their having more beds than patients to fill them, and (2) frail elderly people who were disabled often needed to go to nursing homes far from where they lived. In this chapter, Sharon Begley, science columnist with the *Wall Street Journal*, who has contributed previously to *The Robert Wood Johnson Foundation Anthology*, tells the story of how some thoughtful leaders devised a seemingly simple solution to these two problems: use empty hospital beds for patients needing long-term skilled nursing care.

Begley goes on to describe how the swing-bed idea developed, even over the initial reluctance of federal regulators to make an exception to Medicare regulations, the suspicion with which nursing homes received the idea, and the uncertainty about the level of care a practitioner could offer the occupant of a swing bed. The idea took hold, however; today, more than 60 percent of rural hospitals have swing-bed arrangements.

In retrospect, the swing-bed concept proceeded in an unusually ideal manner: it was tested on a small scale, outcomes were measured, and then the model was slowly expanded to other rural areas. The federal government was involved from the beginning; the Foundation entered as the idea was gathering steam and was able to influence development and help guide the direction it took. As with many service innovations, the Foundation's role was strategic and supportive, representing just one force in a larger national effort.

—ɯ— I̲n early October 1969, Dr. Bruce Walter and three colleagues were driving through eastern Utah on an annual mission: the four state officials were visiting rural hospitals to certify compliance with Medicare standards. Without certification, the hospitals would not be reimbursed for the care they provided to Medicare patients. As these officials drove between Moab and Monticello, they talked about the plight of rural hospitals. Although many were new or renovated, thanks to federal money from the Hill-Burton program, which began in the 1940s, they were struggling financially, because demand for acute, hospital-based care in rural communities just wasn't as strong as many planners had predicted. Nursing homes in those communities, though, were often oversubscribed: they had a high occupancy rate and, often, a long waiting list. Worst off were communities without a nursing home. In Moab, for instance, elderly residents in need of long-term care were typically sent to nursing homes far from where they lived—and that meant they were also far from their doctors, their family, and their friends.

The four officials lobbed ideas back and forth about how Moab might keep its financially beleaguered hospital, which was not only a source of acute health care but also a critical cog in the local economy, and at the same time accommodate the elderly who needed long-term care. Eventually, someone asked: Why not provide nursing home care in empty hospital beds?

At that time, Walter was Utah's director of Medicare services. When he got back to Salt Lake City, he wrote to the regional Medicare office in Denver, laying out the problem. Rural communities faced a shortage of nursing home beds in Medicare-certified skilled nursing facilities, he noted. That reflected the "industry's unwillingness or inability to meet the Medicare certification standards," as well as a paucity of the private pay patients needed to support a skilled nursing facility, Walter said.[1] The shortage of skilled nursing beds—three per thousand people over sixty-five in South Dakota, Texas, and Iowa in the mid-1970s, compared to fifteen per thousand nationally—reflected business pragmatism. In other words, there were too few patients in rural areas to justify expansion. As a result, those facilities that did exist typically had a high occupancy rate and a long waiting list, leaving rural residents, especially elderly ones, with little access to long-term care.

Yet in many of the communities suffering a shortage of nursing home beds, the local hospitals had an oversupply of (or at least were underusing) acute care hospital beds. This reflected a declining population, a physician shortage, and the exodus of patients through referrals to an urban hospital. It might have seemed obvious to provide skilled nursing care in those empty beds, but federal regulations did not allow that. If a hospital wanted to provide intermediate-level care or skilled nursing care, Medicare and Medicaid regulations required doing so in a facility that was physically distinct from acute-care beds. The facility for long-term care could be used for no other purpose and had to provide social services, physical therapy, and social and recreational activities that would help patients remain ambulatory, or become ambulatory and be able to carry out activities of daily life.

Meeting this standard would have meant significant additional cost. Yet the Medicare reimbursement for the skilled nursing care long-term care patients would require was less than that for acute care. Many rural hospitals, especially smaller ones, struggled to meet these requirements; the paperwork threatened to swamp their accounting capability and skilled staff was often insufficient. The "physically distinct" requirement for long-term care facilities thus ended a tradition in community hospitals of caring for both acute and long-term patients. Unable to offer a physically distinct facility for such care, a rural hospital would be unable to offer it at all—just at a time when America's elderly population was increasing and demands for such care were rising.

So two trends—excess acute bed capacity and shortage of extended-care beds in rural areas—crossed, and out of that juncture emerged Bruce Walter's idea. Why not address both, he suggested, by letting rural hospitals fill their empty acute-care beds with long-term care patients? The regional Medicare office agreed, and encouraged Medicare headquarters back East to consider some kind of experimental program. After negotiations that were "more than a little tense," and multiple presentations by Walter to U.S. Senate committees and meetings with Medicare officials, he finally got the answer he was looking for. "We'll see what we can do," Tom Tierney, Medicare's first director, told Walter after an April 1972 meeting.[2]

—ᴍ— The First Swing Beds: Utah, 1973

What Tierney could do, it turned out, was fund a three-year experiment named the Utah Cost Improvement Project, starting in January 1973. It involved twenty-five small rural hospitals in Utah. These hospitals became eligible for Medicare and Medicaid reimbursement for long-term care that they provided in acute-care beds—and the first swing-bed program was under way.

It is worth pausing here to clarify some terminology. From its inception, the swing-bed program has been described as providing "long-term care." There are three types of such care: skilled nursing, intermediate nursing, and custodial. Custodial care includes administering single medications and assisting with such activities of daily living as bathing and getting dressed. Medicare does not cover this. Nor does it cover intermediate-level care—what Marjorie Eddinger of the Centers for Medicare & Medicaid Services (formerly the Health Care Financing Administration) in the Department of Health and Human Services calls "caring for the walking wounded, like changing dressings." What Medicare does cover is "skilled nursing care." This includes injections, intravenous feedings, placing catheters, rehabilitation (speech, physical, and occupational), and the like. It is what participants in the swing-bed program meant by long-term care.

A swing bed does not swing physically. Rather, it swings in the way hospital accountants and medical staff treat the patient occupying it. In a swing-bed program, a patient being treated for an acute condition could remain in the hospital for follow-up long-term care rather than be discharged to a nursing home. She or he would usually stay in the same bed, but the kind of care would be different, and the accountants would bill for it differently. Medicare's reimbursement for services such as x-rays and lab work was based on the hospital's cost for these services. It reimbursed hospitals for skilled nursing care at the Medicaid per-diem rate, covering room, board, and nursing. A hospital received less money from the government for long-term care than for acute-level care, but it was income that would not be received if the patient were discharged to a nursing facility. Moreover, the hospital didn't have to meet the Medicare standards for rehabilitation services, social services, and space for patient activities.

These two provisions—waiver of Medicare standards for long-term care and a novel reimbursement scheme—were crucial to the swing-bed experiment.

All of the participating hospitals must have had fewer than fifty beds and less than 60 percent occupancy in the three previous years.

Yet even in such underused hospitals, the idea of the swing bed was not accepted without reservation. "The administrators were leery from the beginning," says Peter Shaughnessy, of the University of Colorado Health Sciences Center, who led the team that evaluated the swing-bed program. They were suspicious of federal intervention, and most knew next to nothing about long-term care. "At the start, the reaction of the nursing staff was often, 'This kind of care is beneath me; you don't need my special skills,'" Shaughnessy says. The nursing home industry was none too happy, either, figuring that swing beds would steal their patients. Many health planners doubted the wisdom of trying to prop up rural hospitals: if the facilities were operating at such low capacity, the reasoning went, they should be closed, not bailed out with this or any other program. But the greatest concern of all was that the care in swing beds might be substandard; as the hospitals themselves admitted, what did they know about long-term care?

That's what Shaughnessy and his team at the University of Colorado set out to answer. In an evaluation sponsored by the federal government, the Colorado team found, first of all, that long-term care patients loved swing beds: being in a hospital made them feel better cared for, and since they weren't physically moved to a nursing home, the program was much less disruptive than a move to a nursing home would have been. Families loved keeping grandma in her home town and not having to travel to a distant nursing home to see her. Physicians liked swing beds because they could visit their patients more frequently than if they were sent to a nursing home. Administrators and nurses came to like swing beds for satisfying the community's long-term care needs. "That's what I've always liked about the staff at these small rural hospitals," Shaughnessy says. "They were responsive to patients' needs, and they were also very aware of the important place the hospital had in the community, both as an employer and as a symbol. Even though neither the acute-care staff nor the nurses' aides were trained in long-term care, they quickly realized that these patients had different needs, and learned to meet those needs. What turned them around was seeing that their patients really benefited from swing-bed care."

—w— Expanding the Idea: 1976

In 1976, the federal government expanded the trial program in hospital swing beds to 39 hospitals in Texas and 22 in South Dakota and western Iowa, and in 1977 to 22 in central Iowa, until the program encompassed 108 rural hospitals in those four states. As in the original Utah experiment, small rural hospitals (with fewer than fifty beds) would use their beds interchangeably, swinging them between acute care and nursing-home-type care, depending on demand.

Who were the early swing-bed patients? Most were and are female, typically a white widow, seventy-five or older, covered by Medicare. This typical patient was living at home, either alone or with family. A fracture (in 20 percent of cases) or stroke (12 percent) sent her to acute care. In long-term care, she sat in a chair for meals (53 percent of patients), received physical therapy (56 percent), participated in patient activities twice a week or more (41 percent), and received social services weekly (49 percent). After discharge, she returned home to live alone or with relatives, though one in four went to a nursing home. One in ten died while in the swing bed; one in eleven returned to an acute-care bed.[3] They were patients like a seventy-eight-year-old woman at Sierra Vista Hospital in Truth or Consequences, New Mexico, who had chronic obstructive pulmonary disease. She was moved to long-term care for two weeks and then back to acute care (never physically changing beds, of course) when she contracted pneumonia. She went back to long-term care for a month and then back to acute care when she needed increased oxygen therapy.

Once again, the evaluators found that hospital administrators, physicians, nurses, patients, and patients' families were enthusiastic about swing beds.[4] Even nursing home administrators in the community or nearby signed on, with the majority concluding that the swing-bed program should be not only continued but also expanded.

The biggest trouble spot was in quality of care. Some hospital staff members had difficulty switching gears to care for a long-term patient. Partly as a result, "the quality of long-term care provided in swing-bed hospitals was lower than . . . in comparison nursing homes." In particular, the hospitals rated worse not only on such measures as addressing psychosocial problems, which fall outside their usual bailiwick, but even in such chronic-care needs as incontinence, skin condition, depression, loneliness, and isolation. Nursing homes were also better at "social-recreation, therapeutic-mental health, physical and occupational therapies, professional nursing," the evaluators found, as well as in caring for patients requiring basic maintenance and support of their "functional, cognitive, emotional, and social needs." Services were uneven: 53 percent of the swing-bed hospitals offered physical therapy and 36 percent offered social services, while speech therapy, occupational therapy, and patient activities were offered less frequently.

The extent to which the hospitals embraced swing beds also varied wildly, from 8 days of long-term care in one hospital to 3,667 in another. Not surprisingly, perhaps, the evaluators found that "hospitals with lower occupancy rates tended to provide more long-term care than those with higher occupancy rates." The occupancy rates of nursing homes in rural areas hardly budged, however, indicating that swing beds were not substituting for rural nursing home beds but adding to them.

Swing beds were cost-effective, though they were not the revenue gusher that some administrators initially hoped for. "Swing beds were not big profit makers, but they did provide revenue and enable hospitals to keep open and retain staff," Shaughnessy said. Compared to nursing homes, hospital swing beds were better able to provide the near-acute care (rather than chronic care) that most of their patients required. (Someone recovering from hip surgery or requiring an IV would be a near-acute patient.) Physicians visited swing-bed patients more frequently than they did nursing home patients. "Long-term care for the types of patients typically treated in hospital swing beds was adequate and possibly even above average, but . . . chronic care for patients with maintenance and even palliative care needs potentially required improvement," the Colorado evaluators found.[5] The experiment "showed that a hospital's ability to 'swing' beds between acute and long-term care services could satisfy the need in rural communities for both services while maintaining sufficient reimbursement for the hospital," the American Hospital Association concluded in 1982, referring to the 108-hospital program.[6]

The evaluators recommended that the swing-bed program go national. Many rural communities faced an unmet need for long-term care, they argued;

swing beds could be more cost-effective than alternatives such as building more nursing homes; patients and their families benefited from staying near home; and swing beds could shore up rural hospitals financially. A swing-bed program "would be of benefit to rural communities in terms of meeting both long-term care and acute care needs," the evaluation team wrote in 1980. Moreover, swing beds were "a cost-effective means of providing long-term care." The quality of long-term care they offered was considered adequate, and although nursing homes scored better "the discrepancy was not substantial and . . . is likely to disappear over time as the staffs of swing-bed hospitals become familiar with the special problems of the long-term care patient."[7]

—⚶— Swing Beds Go National

The eight-year experiment was deemed enough of a success that in 1980, when Congress passed the Omnibus Budget Reconciliation Act, it included a provision allowing Medicare and Medicaid to pay for swing-bed care in rural hospitals that had fewer than fifty beds. In all, more than twenty-two hundred hospitals were eligible. The Health Care Financing Administration issued implementing regulations in July 1982: it imposed straightforward quality standards (requiring the specialized rehabilitation, patient activities, discharge planning, and other services of skilled nursing facilities) and reimbursement policies (as with the pilot program, routine room, board, and nursing were reimbursed according to the state average Medicaid day rate for skilled nursing facilities, and reimbursement for ancillary services were based on cost).

Coping with Medicare regulations was often difficult for small rural hospitals, and probably for others as well. To make things even more confusing, in March 1983 Medicare began reimbursing hospitals under a "prospective payment system." Rather than reimbursing hospitals on the basis of the number of days they cared for patients and what they did for them, Medicare now reimbursed hospitals according to a patient's diagnostic-related group, or DRG. A hospital that kept, say, a hip-replacement patient for ten days would get the same reimbursement as one that kept him for nine. This was an incentive to discharge patients as soon as possible—and, according to critics, in some cases sooner than was reasonable. Such patients seemed more likely to receive the postacute care they needed in a swing bed, which had a stronger medical orientation, than in a nursing home bed.

The change in reimbursement also increased the controversy swirling around swing beds. The nursing home industry charged that hospitals were using swing beds to do an end run around the prospective payment system. (Medicare will pay for only this number of days for my hip fracture patient? No problem, from that day on I'll have Accounting say she's in a swing bed.) There were even concerns that swing beds might allow double dipping, with hospitals being reimbursed twice for services that the prospective payment system was intended to cover. According to this argument, the services that swing patients received—caring for postsurgical wounds, for instance—were included in the hospital's DRG.

Although the new Medicare prospective payment system slowed adoption of swing-bed programs as small rural hospitals sorted out the incentives and the disincentives, by 1984 it was clear that the prospective payment system offered incentives for rural hospitals to provide swing-bed care.[8] The number of participating hospitals grew steadily: 149 at the end of 1983 to 771 (out of an estimated 1,600 eligible rural hospitals in thirty-nine states) at the end of 1985 and 1,207 by August 1989.

—ᴠᴠ— The Robert Wood Johnson Foundation Swing-Bed Program: 1981

Starting a swing-bed program requires meeting the care and administrative requirements that Congress and the Health Care Financing Agency imposed. The complexity of the reimbursement procedures created management problems for many small rural hospitals. Moreover, directors and staff members of many of those hospitals resisted the idea that an acute-care hospital should become a nursing home. As a result of these and other barriers, by the end of the four-state federal demonstration a third of the eligible hospitals had elected not to participate. Although Congress had changed federal reimbursement mechanisms, it had done little or nothing to address such issues.

The Robert Wood Johnson Foundation already had a vibrant program in rural health care, recalls senior program officer Nancy Barrand: "This seemed like the next logical step in our efforts to help small rural hospitals and the communities they served." So in April 1981, the Foundation launched a national demonstration program called the Rural Hospital Program of Extended-Care Services. The $6.5 million program provided funding for five state hospital associations and twenty-six small rural hospitals in those states to convert acute-care beds to swing beds. The goals, explained Thomas Gregg, a Robert Wood Johnson Foundation program officer, and Robert Blendon, a Foundation vice president, were to improve patient access to long-term care and help financially precarious rural hospitals, and do it all in a cost-effective way. To accomplish all this, the Foundation would promote swing beds by establishing models of how a small rural hospital with excess acute care beds in an area that also had a nursing home shortage could provide high-quality long-term care.[9]

How? By raising awareness of the program, showing hospitals how to adopt it successfully, developing technical expertise in the hospitals and state associations, and having participants share what they learned.[10] Hospitals could use the grants from The Robert Wood Johnson Foundation for training, to pay for replacements of those being trained, to pay for those providing specialized services like physical therapy, and to obtain equipment. They could organize training sessions on billing Medicare and Medicaid for swing-bed stays, since negotiating the shoals of Medicare reimbursement was no easy matter. Grantees could also offer educational programs in gerontology, to help nurses deal with what, to many, was the more frustrating and less interesting work (compared to acute care) of caring for the chronically ill. Training was crucial, since, as the Foundation officers gently noted, "hospital staff may be reluctant to change their methods of operation."

One of the program's chief elements was to help grantee hospitals narrow the gap between the services they offered in swing beds and those that nursing homes offered in long-term care beds. Hospitals offered swing-bed patients fewer social and recreational services, therapeutic and mental health services, and physical and occupational therapy services than did high-quality nursing homes. There was genuine concern among Foundation officers that the hospital-based long-term care was inadequate in these areas and had to be improved. Finally, but not least, the Foundation's program had the ambitious intent of overcoming reluctance to adopt the swing-bed approach by enhancing the medical, administrative, and financial capacity to deliver care.

"What the Foundation did was immensely clever," evaluator Peter Shaughnessy said. "They took a program we knew something about, and as national implementation was going forward they said, 'Let's be sure it's done well.' Without these grants, swing beds would not have brought the widespread benefits for so many patients that they did. The education and training that resulted from the grants was exactly what was needed. They provided a template."

To direct the program, the Foundation named Tony Kovner of New York University's Robert F. Wagner Graduate School of Public Service and a former rural hospital administrator.

As the swing-bed program was launched, hopes were high. In a memo recommending the grant program, Gregg and Blendon noted that if every rural hospital participated in the swing-bed program, "between three-quarters of a million and two million days of long-term care would be provided in rural hospital 'swing-beds,'" a 10 percent increase in the availability of such care in rural areas, and the program would offer rural residents "an instant alternative to some of the smaller and less adequate proprietary nursing homes."[11]

The Robert Wood Johnson Foundation program got off to a rocky start, however. Despite intensive training, many hospitals found that nurses resented the extra workload and, inappropriately and expensively, provided the same high level of care to swing-bed patients that they did to acute-care patients. Because of inexperience and lacking local resources such as physical therapists, many of the grantee hospitals were unable to offer enough high-quality patient activity programs. In one New Mexico hospital, two patients who were admitted to long-term care in swing beds stayed only a few days, since the nursing staff refused to take care of them and the director of nursing did not support the program. Even where hospitals did a good job, as in Kansas, there were glitches: hospitals were denied reimbursement because of confusion about the definition of skilled-level care.

Even with these startup problems, the number of patient days in the swing beds rose steadily, from 1,526 in 1983 to 8,522 in 1984 and 10,221 in 1985. Over the same period, patient-days in acute-care beds fell 20 percent, suggesting that swing beds had a stabilizing effect on the hospitals.[12]

—ᴡ— Assessing the Swing-Bed Program

Any assessment of the swing-bed program needs to be clear about whether it is addressing the program's value to the patient or its value to the hospital. On the first count, both those running the program and those evaluating it found swing beds a success. Tony Kovner, the program director, and Hila Richardson, the deputy director, found that swing beds increased access to long-term care for rural residents, especially those with intense medical needs. More residents stayed in their community for such care than did those where swing beds were unavailable. Compared with nursing homes, swing beds excelled in several areas. They made possible a smooth continuum of care from initial hospital admission through discharge to home or nursing home. Swing-bed patients had easier access to such medical services as respiratory therapy and lab tests.[13]

Perhaps their care improved simply because they were allowed to recover near home, where family and friends could be involved in their care.[14] Peter Shaughnessy was particularly impressed that "critical ingredients of long-term care that were often missing in other settings were beginning to occur in swing-bed settings."[15] In particular, physicians became more involved in long-term care. Certain kinds of rehabilitation as well as skilled nursing care were more available than in a nursing home. Care for patients segueing from acute care to long-term care was better coordinated. These differences from traditional long-term care accounted for the swing-bed program's success.

Although the quality of care got mostly good marks, there were some stumbling blocks. The first was that caring for a patient in a swing bed is significantly different from caring for a patient in a traditional hospital bed. As a result, the medical staff had to change its focus from diagnosis-centered, doctor-dominated, acute care to the nursing-centered, multidimensional needs of the long-term-care patient. There was no question that the old mold of hospital care needed to be broken when it came to the swing-bed patient. At Cedar County Memorial Hospital in El Dorado Springs, Missouri, staff members learned not to do everything for the patient, as they did for those in acute care, but to assist (or simply stand by) while the swing-bed patients fed and dressed themselves. The staff involved the family in a patient's care, encouraging relatives to come at meal-time and bath time to lend a hand, and to stay after visiting hours to help the patient get ready to sleep. At all the hospitals, the staff learned a new way of work-ing: physicians did not necessarily visit swing-bed patients daily, as they typically do acute-care patients. Nurses carried out assessment and referral for swing-bed services and made recommendations for long-term care to the physician rather than the other way around.

Not surprisingly, perhaps, hospitals did better at things they were used to doing: meeting basic medical and nursing needs, and providing diagnostic and lab tests. Tasks such as making an activity available for patients and performing a functional assessment presented more problems, and hospital staff members generally did not carry them out as well as nursing home staff people did. In large part, this difference reflected the low number of swing-bed patients. It's one thing to organize bridge games, music recitals, crafts activities, and outings for a score of patients in a nursing home, but quite another to do so for the three patients in your swing beds. The staff time per patient soars, and it's tough to motivate staff members to shift gears when they typically have only three to five swing-bed patients. When there's an acute-care patient in this bed, an aide may feed her. But the aide has to sit patiently while the swing-bed patient right next door feeds herself. Finally, some 40 percent of swing-bed patients stayed fewer than ten days, so the difficulty of long-term assessment left many staff members frustrated. Swing beds "lack the critical mass of patients to carry out successful patient activities or to justify hiring some specialized staff," concluded Joshua Wiener, a Brook-ings Institution researcher.[16]

An unforeseen problem arose from the fact that swing beds are not physically distinct or separate. Tension sometimes arose: the patient in the acute-care bed received more nursing than the person in the swing bed beside him, causing resentment by the swing-bed patient (and her family). Why is Grandma getting less help and care than her roommate? The American Hospital Association, or AHA, which cosponsored the swing-bed program, concluded, "When mismanaged, swing beds can induce negative side effects . . . reducing the quality of both the acute and long-term care available to the community and having a detrimental effect on hospital finances and work relationships."[17]

Although "work relationships" mattered, the AHA made it clear that the finances of swing beds concerned it most. The association exhorted members to use available beds as acute-care beds whenever possible; if a hospital has so many swing-bed patients (requiring skilled nursing care) that it has to turn away acute-care patients, the bottom line suffers (since reimbursement rates are less). Even hiring staff members for skilled nursing-care patients is financially problematic, the AHA warned.[18] If such patients "are given the same level of nursing care as acute patients, the income statement is again threatened," the association continued. It exhorted hospitals to get relatives to lend a hand feeding and dressing patients.

Unexpectedly, swing beds benefited hospital staff in some ways. The presence of specialized professionals and the chance to learn about the needs of the elderly made hospital staff members more aware of the rehabilitative and psychosocial needs of all patients, particularly elderly acute patients. Also, the need to provide swing-bed patients with physical, occupational, and speech therapy, as well as social services and discharge planning, made these processes available to acute care patients too. Acute patients often availed themselves of social programs. Also, swing beds let nurses take more responsibility for patient care, and physicians less, offering a better chance for professional development. Swing beds were even good for the bottom line, yielding some 8 percent of total inpatient revenue. This covered the cost of the program and, in the majority of hospitals, reduced the deficit or increased a surplus.[19]

Swing beds were still not stealing patients from nursing homes, but not for the reason their proponents expected. By 1985, it was clear that swing beds were serving primarily near-acute care patients. Their "long-term care" wasn't very long; recall that the average length of stay for all swing-bed patients was twenty days. Compared to a nursing home patient, a swing-bed patient was more likely to be recovering from surgery, to have an IV catheter, and to have had a recent stroke or hip fracture or heart attack with congestive heart failure. "In rural communities, swing-bed hospitals had gravitated predominantly toward providing near-acute care and were not competing with nursing homes for more traditional chronic care patients who required maintenance and palliative care," Shaughnessy concluded.[20] Hospital swing-bed programs, in other words, were playing to their strength—something that continues today. Swing beds, as Kovner and his colleagues noted, seem to "work best for patients who require short-stay, medically intensive services in small, rural hospitals that can recruit the necessary specialized staff. It is not a program for all post-acute patients, particularly long-stay patients."[21]

That did not always placate nursing home operators, however. Throughout the 1980s, swing-bed programs still faced opposition from the industry, which in some states lobbied hard to require a hospital to be licensed as a nursing home before being allowed to operate swing beds.

—⟋⟍— Reflecting on the Swing-Bed Concept

Are swing beds cost-effective? As long as the hospital has surplus physical capacity and staff, the answer is yes: the marginal cost of providing long-term care in a swing bed runs some 45 percent less than it would have been to provide that care by building a nursing home, noted Joshua Wiener of Brookings.[22] If an existing home has excess beds, however, or if it can easily add beds, then that option is cheaper than swing beds. "The swing-bed program cannot, on its own, save a failing hospital," a 1985 conference sponsored by The Robert Wood Johnson Foundation program and the Texas Hospital Association concluded, "but it can provide revenue to help a hospital survive."[23] By the mid-1980s, hospitals with swing-bed programs were gaining, on average, between eight and ten dollars a day per patient under the program. The ancillary care cost hospitals about twenty dollars a day per patient, but brought in some thirty-two dollars in daily revenue. Although some hospitals groused that they should be reimbursed at a higher rate, the financial set-up cannot have been too bad; by the mid-1980s, more than half the eligible hospitals were participating. Although revenues typically exceeded costs in hospital swing beds, the programs nevertheless saved money for Medicare and Medicaid. "It appears that the swing-bed program has paid for itself under Medicare by lowering costs through reductions in rehospitalizations and physician reimbursement after discharge," Peter Shaughnessy observed in 1991.[24]

By that year, swing-bed programs were "providing patients with demonstrably higher-quality care than they were likely to receive elsewhere, minimizing burdens on family members, and helping to insure the survival of rural health care institutions," wrote Bruce Vladeck, then president of the United Hospital Fund of New York and former head of the federal Health Care Financing Administration. But if the outcome was noteworthy, so was the process. Swing beds evolved "from an initial though preliminary experimentation, to more systematic testing, and then through successive iterations of modest expansion accompanied by thorough evaluation," Vladeck noted—the way innovative health care programs are supposed to arise, perhaps, but rarely do. He elaborated: "An innovative idea was tested on a small scale; the apparent success of that innovation was followed by somewhat larger tests of the idea with minor variants, and those tests were closely monitored; new policy, based largely on the results of those tests, was adopted."[25]

Swing beds have remained a rural program. Periodically throughout the 1990s, advocates of swing beds approached the Health Care Financing Administration to argue that they be expanded to urban hospitals. City hospitals, however, could not make the case that they were providing a service for which the elderly would otherwise have to travel to a distant facility (after all, most cities have lots of nursing homes). In rural areas, however, swing beds have taken hold. In 2001, "about 63 percent of rural hospitals, about one thousand, had swing bed agreements," says Ira Moscovice, professor and director of the University of Minnesota Rural Health Research Center. "Swing beds accounted for about 20 percent of the patient-days in these hospitals, or eight hundred days per hospital. Just as in the beginning of the program, swing beds won't make or break a rural hospital, but they do make a difference on the margin—the difference between a hospital being a little bit in the hole to balancing its books. Swing beds remain an important program for rural hospitals."

Notes

1. Richardson, H., Wiener, J. M., and Kovner, A. R. "Swing-Beds: Current Experience and Future Directions." (Unpublished report prepared for The Robert Wood Johnson Foundation) 1986.

2. Shaughnessy, P. *Shaping Policy for Long-Term Care: Learning from the Effectiveness of Hospital Swing Beds.* Chicago: Health Administration Press, 1991.

3. Richardson, Wiener, and Kovner (1986).

4. Tynan, E., and others. "An Evaluation of Swing-Bed Experiments to Provide Long-Term Care in Rural Hospitals." (Health Care Financing Grants and Contracts Report.) HCFA, 1980.

5. Shaughnessy (1991).

6. American Hospital Association. "Curing the Ills of Hospital Underutilization: The Swing-Bed Treatment and Its Side Effects." *Small or Rural Hospital Report,* Jan.–Feb. 1982.

7. Tynan and others (1980).

8. Shaughnessy (1991).

9. Gregg, T., and Blendon, R. "A Program to Aid Small Rural Hospitals in Providing Long-Term Care Utilizing the 'Swing-Bed' Concept." (Internal Robert Wood Johnson Foundation report, unpublished) 1981.

10. Wiener, J. "Introduction and Summary." In J. Wiener (ed.), *Swing Beds: Assessing Flexible Health Care in Rural Communities.* Washington, D.C.: Brookings, 1987.

11. Gregg and Blendon (1981).

12. Kovner, A., and Richardson, H. "The Robert Wood Johnson Demonstration Program." In Wiener (1987).

13. Kovner and Richardson (1987).

14. Wiener (1987).

15. Shaughnessy (1991).

16. Wiener (1987).

17. American Hospital Association (1982).

18. American Hospital Association (1982).

19. Richardson, Wiener, and Kovner (1986).

20. Shaughnessy (1991).

21. Richardson, Wiener, and Kovner (1986).

22. Wiener (1987).

23. "A Summary from a Conference on Swing Beds." Conference sponsored by the Rural Hospital Program of Extended Care and the Texas Hospital Association, September 23–24, 1985, San Antonio, Texas.
24. Shaughnessy (1991).
25. Vladeck, B. "The Meaning of the Swing-Bed Experience." In Wiener (1987).

—ɯ— The Editors

Stephen L. Isaacs, J.D., is the president of Health Policy Associates in San Francisco. A former professor of public health at Columbia University and founding director of its Development Law and Policy Program, he has written extensively for professional and popular audiences. His book *The Consumer's Legal Guide to Today's Health Care* was reviewed as "the single best guide to the health care system in print today." His articles have been widely syndicated and have appeared in law reviews and health policy journals. He also provides technical assistance internationally on health law, civil society, and social policy. A graduate of Brown University and Columbia Law School, Isaacs served as vice president of International Planned Parenthood's Western Hemisphere Region, practiced health law, and spent four years in Thailand as a program officer for the U.S. Agency for International Development.

James R. Knickman, Ph.D., is vice president for research and evaluation at The Robert Wood Johnson Foundation. He oversees a range of grants and national programs supporting research and policy analysis to better understand forces that can improve health status and delivery of health care. In addition, he is in charge of developing formal evaluations of national programs supported by the Foundation. He has also played a leadership role in developing grant-making strategy in the area of chronic illness during his seven years at the Foundation. During the 1999-2000 academic year, he held a Regents' Lectureship at the University of California, Berkeley. Previously, Knickman was on the faculty of the Robert Wagner Graduate School of Public Service at New York University. At NYU, he was the founding director of a universitywide research center focused on urban health care. His publications include research on a range of health care topics, with particular emphasis on issues related to financing and delivering long-term care. He has served on numerous health-related advisory committees at the state and local levels and spent a year working at New York City's Office of Management and Budget. Currently, he serves on the board of trustees of Robert Wood Johnson University Hospital and chairs the board's committee overseeing construction of a new Children's Hospital in New Brunswick. He completed his undergraduate work at Fordham University and received his doctorate in public policy analysis from the University of Pennsylvania.

—⚅— The Contributors

Joseph Alper has been a science and health care writer for twenty-two years. During that time, he has served as a contributing correspondent for *Science* and as a contributing editor of *Nature Biotechnology* and *Self* magazines. He has also written for a variety of publications, including the *Atlantic Monthly, Harper's,* the *New York Times,* the *Washington Post,* and *Health Magazine,* and has written numerous policy documents for the National Institutes of Health and the National Academy of Science. Alper has won several national writing awards, including the American Chemical Society's Grady/Stack Award for career achievements in science writing and two national writing awards from the American Psychological Association. Alper has also taught journalism and writing at the University of Wisconsin-Madison, Johns Hopkins University, the University of Minnesota, and Colorado State University. He graduated from the University of Illinois-Urbana and received master's of science degrees in biochemistry and agricultural journalism from the University of Wisconsin-Madison.

Sharon Begley was a senior editor at *Newsweek,* where she covered science since 1977. She has won numerous awards for her journalism, including the Clarion Award from Women in Communications, the Distinguished Achievement Award from the Educational Press Association of America, the Global Award for Media Excellence from the Population Institute, and the Wilbur Award from the National Religious Public Relations Council. She is now the science columnist at the *Wall Street Journal.*

Paul Brodeur was a staff writer at the *New Yorker* for nearly forty years. During that time, he alerted the nation to the public health hazard posed by asbestos, to depletion of the ozone layer by chlorofluorocarbons, and to the harmful effects

273

of microwave radiation and power-frequency electromagnetic fields. His work has been acknowledged with a National Magazine Award and the Journalism Award of the American Association for the Advancement of Science. The United Nations Environment Program has named him to its Global 500 Roll of Honour for outstanding environmental achievements.

Ethan Bronner is the assistant editorial page editor of the *New York Times.* From 1999 through 2001, he was the paper's education editor. He came to the *New York Times* in 1997 as a national correspondent and reported on trends in higher education and grades K–12. From 1985 until 1997, he was with the *Boston Globe,* where he served as Middle East correspondent, based in Jerusalem, and a Supreme Court and legal affairs correspondent in Washington, D.C. He began his journalistic career at Reuters in 1980 and reported from London, Madrid, and Brussels. Bronner is the author of *Battle for Justice: How the Bork Nomination Shook America,* which was chosen by the New York Public Library as one of the twenty-five best books of 1989. He received a B.A. in letters from Wesleyan University and an M.S. from Columbia University's School of Journalism.

David C. Colby, Ph.D., is a senior program officer at the Robert Wood Johnson Foundation. He serves as team leader for the Coverage Team and is a member of the Supportive Services Team. He is also the program officer for the Scholars in Health Policy Research and Investigator Awards in Health Policy Research programs. He came to The Robert Wood Johnson Foundation in January 1998 after nine years of service with the Medicare Payment Advisory Commission and the Physician Payment Review Commission, most recently as deputy director. Prior to that he was with the University of Maryland, where he was associate professor in the policy sciences graduate program and coordinator of the Master's of Policy Sciences Program. Colby was a Robert Wood Johnson Faculty Fellow in Health Care Finance, serving in the Congressional Budget Office. Earlier he was dean of freshmen and assistant dean at Williams College and held faculty positions at Williams College and State University College at Buffalo. His published research has focused on Medicaid and Medicare, media coverage of AIDS, and various topics in political science. He was an associate editor of the *Journal of Health Politics, Policy and Law* from 1995 to 2002. He received his doctorate in political science from the University of Illinois, M.A. from Ohio University, and B.A. from Ohio Wesleyan University.

Digby Diehl is a writer, literary collaborator, and television, print, and Internet journalist. Recently honored with the Jack Smith Award from the Friends of the Pasadena Public Library, his book credits include *Angel on My Shoulder,* the autobiography of singer Natalie Cole; *The Million Dollar Mermaid,* the autobiography of MGM star Esther Williams; *Tales from the Crypt,* the history of the popular comic book, movie, and television series; and *A Spy for All Seasons,* the autobiography of former CIA officer Duane Clarridge. For eleven years, Diehl was the literary correspondent for ABC-TV's "Good Morning America" and was recently the book editor for the "Home Page" show on MSNBC. He continues to appear regularly on the morning news on KTLA. Previously the entertainment editor for KCBS television in Los Angeles, he was a writer for the Emmys and for the soap opera "Santa Barbara," book editor of the *Los Angeles Herald Examiner,* editor-in-chief of art book publisher Harry N. Abrams, and the founding book editor of the *Los Angeles Times Book Review.* Diehl holds an M.A. in theatre from UCLA and a B.A. in American studies from Rutgers University, where he was a Henry Rutgers Scholar. He is presently collaborating with Coretta Scott King on her memoirs.

Susan B. Garland was a Washington correspondent for twelve years for *Business Week.* Her beats included social policy, the White House, and legal affairs. As social policy reporter, she wrote on a range of health topics, including the uninsured, Medicare, long-term care, attempts by business to control costs through managed care, and government reform efforts. Since the end of 1999, she has been a freelance writer, and her articles on health care, personal finance, and other areas have appeared in *Business Week,* the *Washington Post, Modern Maturity, Parents,* and *Martha Stewart Living.* In 1999, she won an Easter Seals EDI (Equality, Dignity and Independence) Award for her coverage on persons with disabilities. She holds a B.A. from Colgate University, where she was elected to Phi Beta Kappa.

Paul Mantell, in addition to his work for The Robert Wood Johnson Foundation, is a spokesman, writer, actor, educator, and songwriter. With co-author Avery Hart, he has created more than one hundred popular novels for young adults, including dozens of Nancy Drew, Hardy Boys, and Bobbsey Twin mysteries for Simon and Schuster, many of them best-sellers. Additionally, he has written several award-winning works of nonfiction for families and schools, including *Boredom Busters, Kids Garden, Pyramids!, Ancient Greece, Knights and Castles,* and *Kids Make Music.* He has also penned award-winning audio books, plays, songs, and film scripts. Currently, he is the author of Matt Christopher sports books for children 8–12. In addition to his performances on National Public Radio's *In the Dark,* his narrative skills and character acting have delighted thousands of children who have listened to his work on audio cassettes and CDs. As co-creator of the *New Living Newspaper,* Mantell has written and performed in several original shows that dramatize news events and public issues. The *New Living Newspaper* has been personally recognized by Walter Cronkite and favorably reviewed by NBC-TV, the *New York Times*, and others.

Carolyn Newbergh is a Northern California writer who has covered health care trends and policy issues for more than twenty years. Her freelance work has appeared in numerous print and online publications. As a reporter for the *Oakland Tribune,* she wrote articles on health care delivery for the poor as well as emergency room violence, AIDS, and the impact of crack cocaine on the children of addicts. She was also an investigative reporter for the *Tribune*, winning prestigious honors for a series on how consultants intentionally cover up earthquake hazards in California.

C. Tracy Orleans, Ph.D., is senior scientist at The Robert Wood Johnson Foundation. She is responsible for a range of grants and national programs supporting research, programs, and evaluations that focus on translating research into practice and policy in the areas of tobacco control, health and behavior, and chronic disease management. She has played a leadership role in developing grant-making strategy in the area of tobacco-dependence treatment and in the Foundation's efforts to promote adoption of healthy behaviors, especially physical activity. A clinical and health psychologist, she is currently an adjunct professor in the Department of Psychiatry at the University of Medicine and Dentistry of New Jersey. Prior to joining the Foundation's professional staff in 1995, Orleans served as vice president for research and development, Johnson & Johnson Applied Behavioral Technologies, director of tobacco control research at the Fox Chase Cancer Center, and assistant professor of medical psychology and psychiatry at Duke University Medical Center. She has been principal investigator or co-principal investigator on twenty NIH and other research grants and has served on numerous national behavioral-medicine and tobacco-control panels and committees. She has authored or co-authored more than 150 publications; contributed to numerous Surgeon General reports on tobacco; and co-edited, with John Slade, the first medical text on treatment of nicotine addiction. She currently serves on the U.S. Preventive Services Task Force and the Cessation Subcommittee of the Surgeon General's Interagency Committee on Smoking and Health, chairs the Tobacco Cessation Scientific Advisory Panel for the American Legacy Foundation, and serves as past president of the Society of Behavioral Medicine.

Renie Schapiro has an extensive background in health writing and policy. She was a reporter for the *London Sunday Times* and *Time* magazine and editor of *The New Physician* magazine and the *Kennedy Institute of Ethics Journal.* She has published in major medical journals and lay publications. She is co-editor of three books. She was also speechwriter and policy advisor to FDA Commissioner David Kessler and a research associate with the President's Commission on Ethical Problems in Medicine and Biomedical Research. She has taught health policy and bioethics at Yale University and the University of Wisconsin-Madison. She was a special communications officer at The Robert Wood Johnson Foundation and over the past several years has been a consultant to the Foundation, working closely with its president, Steven Schroeder, on papers on health policy and philanthropy. She has an M.P.H from Yale University and a B.A. from the University of Minnesota.

Steven A. Schroeder, M.D., is president and chief executive officer of The Robert Wood Johnson Foundation. A graduate of Stanford University and Harvard Medical School, he trained in internal medicine at the Harvard Medical Service of the Boston City Hospital, in epidemiology as a member of the Epidemic Intelligence Service of the Communicable Diseases Center, and in public health at the Harvard Center for Community Health and Medical Care. He served as an instructor in medicine at Harvard, assistant and associate professor of medicine and health care sciences at George Washington University, and associate professor and professor of medicine at the University of California, San Francisco (UCSF). At both George Washington University and UCSF, he was founding medical director of a university-sponsored health maintenance organization, and at UCSF he founded its Division of General Internal Medicine. While he was the Foundation president, Schroeder continued to practice general internal medicine on a part-time basis at The Robert Wood Johnson Medical School. He has more than 235 publications to his credit. He has served on a number of editorial boards, including (at present) the *New England Journal of Medicine,* and is a member of the boards of the International Advisory Review Committee for the Goldman School of Medicine; Ben Gurion University of Negev, Israel; the American Legacy Foundation; and the Harvard University Board of Overseers. He has received honorary doctorates from Rush University, Boston University, the University of Massachusetts, the Medical College of Wisconsin, and Georgetown University. He retires at the end of 2002, and, as of January 1, 2003, will become Distinguished Professor of Health and Health Care at the University of California, San Francisco.

Irene M. Wielawski is a health care journalist with 20 years experience on daily newspapers, including the *Providence Journal-Bulletin* and the *Los Angeles Times*, where she was a member of the investigations team. She has written extensively on problems of access to care among the poor and uninsured, and other socioeconomic issues in American medicine. From 1994 through 2000, Wielawski—with a research grant from The Robert Wood Johnson Foundation—tracked the experiences of the medically uninsured in twenty-five states following the demise of President Clinton's health reform plan. Other projects in health care journalism since then include helping to develop a pediatric medicine program for public television. Wielawski has been a finalist for the Pulitzer Prize for medical reporting, among other solo honors. She is a founder and former director of the Association of Health Care Journalists, and a graduate of Vassar College.

—⚬— Index

~ຫຼ~Table of Contents
To Improve Health and Health Care 1997

–ᴡ–Table of Contents

To Improve Health and Health Care 1998–1999

–ɯ–Table of Contents
To Improve Health and Health Care 2000

—ɯɯ—Table of Contents
To Improve Health and Health Care 2001

—m—Table of Contents

To Improve Health and Health Care VolumeV